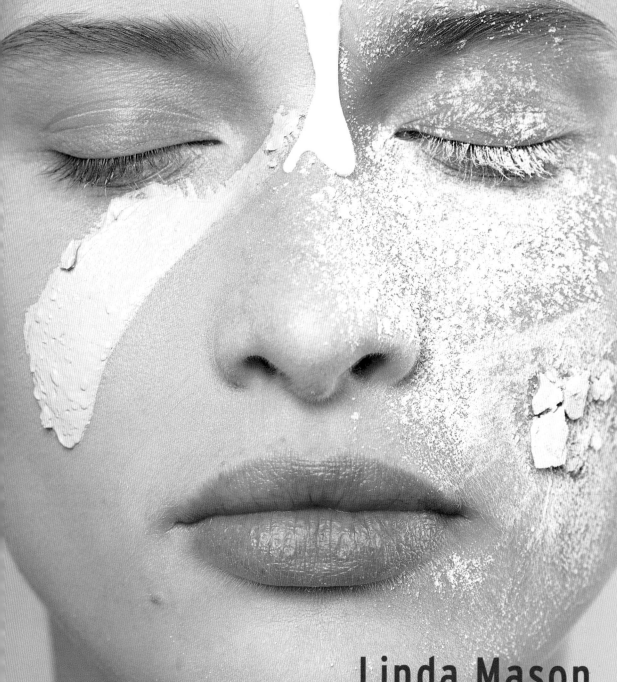

makeup
THE ART OF BEAUTY

Linda Mason

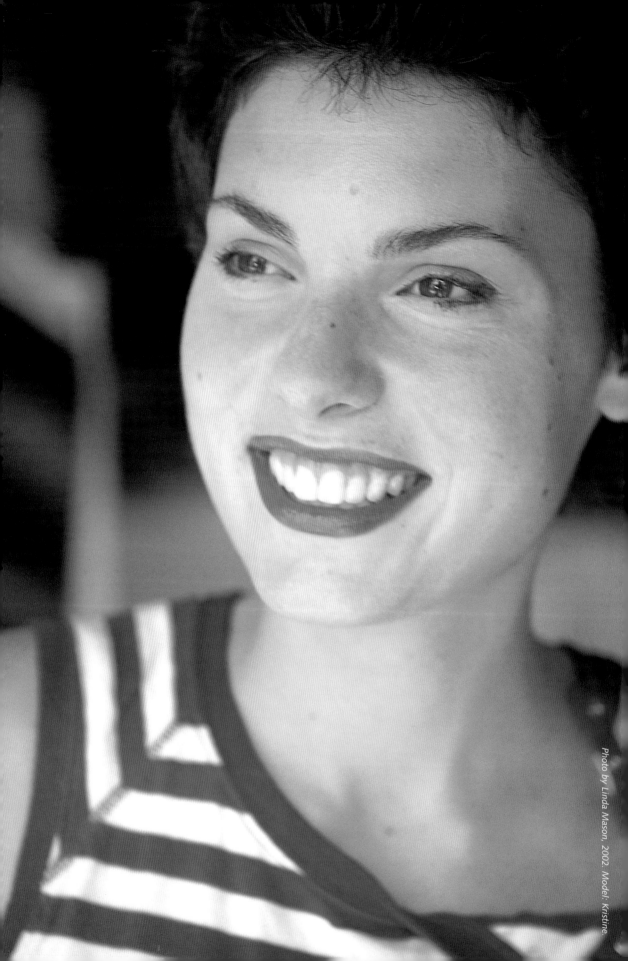

Photo by Linda Mason, 2002. Model: Kristine.

make up
THE ART OF BEAUTY

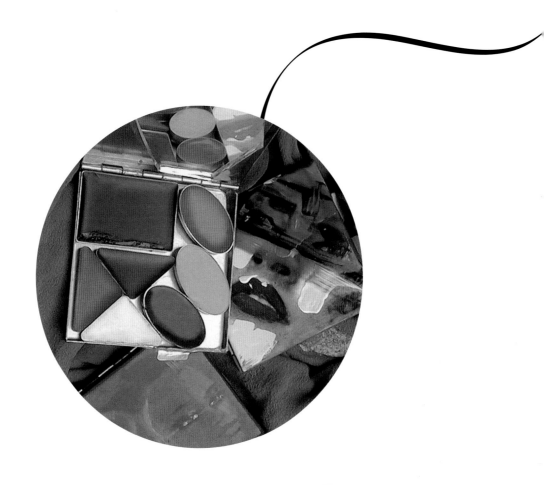

Linda Mason

WATSON-GUPTILL PUBLICATIONS / NEW YORK

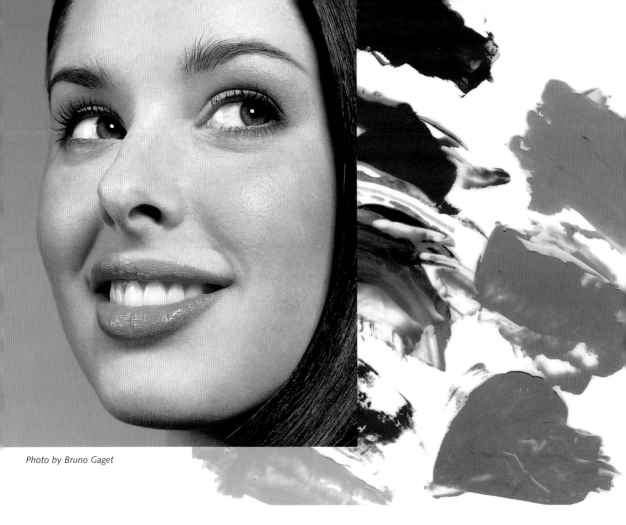

Photo by Bruno Gaget

First published in 2003 by Watson-Guptill Publications,
Nielsen Business Media, a division of The Nielsen Company
770 Broadway, New York, NY 10003
www.watsonguptill.com

Senior Acquisitions Editor: Victoria Craven
Editor: Elizabeth Wright
Design: Margo Mooney, www.pinkdesigninc.com
Production Manager: Sal Destro

Library of Congress Cataloging-in-Publication Data is available from the Library of Congress.
Library of Congress Control Number: 2007920748

Printed in China

First printing, 2003
First paperback printing, 2007

1 2 3 4 5 6 7 8 9 / 08 07

acknowledgments

Many thanks to Senior Acquisitions Editor Victoria Craven for choosing to do this book and for putting together such an incredible team for me to work with. My editor Elizabeth Wright, designers Margo Mooney and Georgia Rucker of Pink Design, Inc., and Production Manager Ellen Greene.

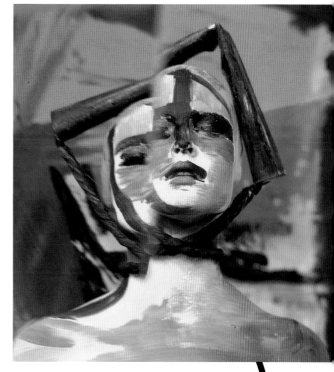

Photo by Matthew Rolston.

The making of this book has allowed me to revisit my life and reconnect with the wonderful and talented people with whom I have been fortunate enough to work. The response from the photographers with whom I have worked during my career was encouraging and overwhelmingly generous. I thank those who so graciously allowed me to use their photographs, as well as those who responded equally generously but whose work was not ultimately included.

Many thanks also to the models and celebrities in these photos for their generous response and for allowing me to use their images. My apologies to those whom I was not able to contact, and to any stylists, art directors, or hair stylists I may not have credited but who have also contributed to the photos.

My agent Jayne Rockmill, whose belief in me, like a rock, was so strong it carried me through.

My daughter Daisy and husband Gene for all their love and support.

Staci Smith, Meghan Hines, Julie Birns, and Nina Allen for their assistance.

A special thanks to Camryn Manheim, Joan Jett, John Galliano, and John Sahag.

To Paulina Poriskova for her timeless beauty and generosity, and to Felicia Rogawska Milewicz for her steadfast support and friendship.

Finally, thanks to the legendary Barbara Daly, whose use of color in the makeup field inspired my first makeup.

contents

Paul Sunday (lips and eyes).

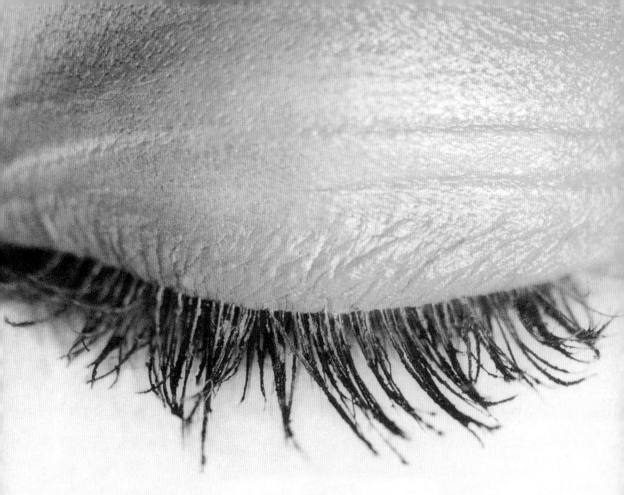

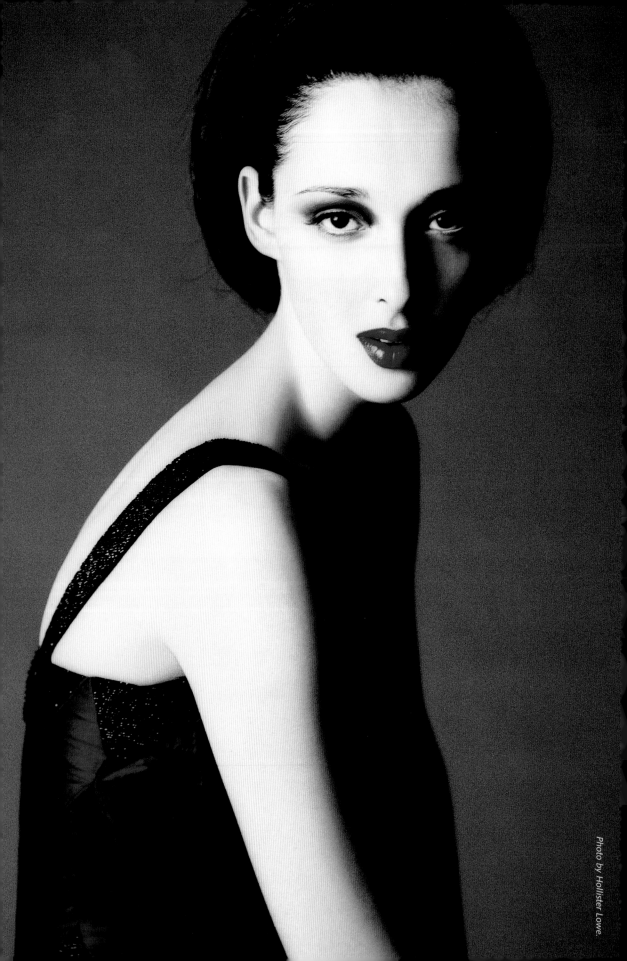

foreword

Linda Mason is one of the most creative makeup artists I have come across in my career. A true makeup artist, Linda always surpasses expectations and takes makeup farther than I could have imagined. Like a real artist, she is fearless, takes risks, expands the parameters, and will always surprise and delight you. She has that true creative element— the ability to surprise—which is so, so important in art but deceptively difficult to achieve.

Linda is and has been known as the "Queen of Color" in the fashion industry for decades. Her makeup style is very recognizable— sometimes subtle, one can always distinguish it by the lips or the eyes or the shape of the mouth. It's the feeling and color that give her away: Her use of color is amazing.

She has inspired many now very successful makeup artists and taught them very generously over the years. We met in Paris in 1982, when I first noticed something unique about her makeup.

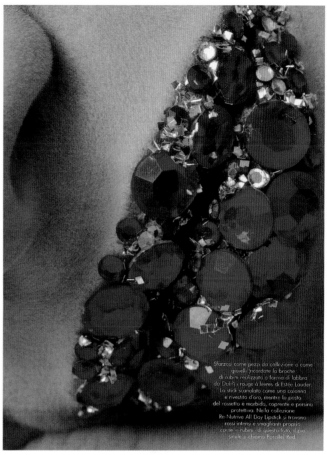

Sfarzosi come pezzi da collezione o come gioielli incordate la broche di rubini realizzata a forma di labbra da Dalì?) i rouge à lèvres di Estée Lauder. Lo stick scanalato come una colonna e rivestito d'oro, mentre la posta del rossetto è morbida, coprente e persino protettiva. Nella collezione Re-Nutriv All Day Lipstick si trovano rossi intensi e smaglianti proprio come i rubini - di questa foto, il più simile si chiama Parallel Red.

Photo by Art Kane.

She has a wonderful approach to creative teamwork. Linda really explores the face as her canvas; she brings out the best in a woman's beauty and does not try to force the same look on everyone. I have also found her to be a great human being at every stage of her career, which has had its ups and downs. She has real talent that has transcended everything, and she has never let ego get in her way.

Linda has good energy, which is very important for someone who is touching other people, and she always exhausts all possibilities. I believe the value of her makeup is better than Prozac. Makeup is a great indulgence that women should give to themselves. We are all forced to be very visually oriented in today's society, and makeup's visual effect—what makeup can *do*—is magical. It's instant gratification. Makeup can not only make you more beautiful on the outside, but can also bring out inner beauty, engendering a sense of self-respect and high self-esteem; at times, it can even make you feel younger.

Women have worn makeup for thousands of years. In this book, Linda details the past century of some of makeup's outstanding trends, from the 1920s through the 1990s to today. Makeup has an interesting past. Linda now transforms makeup in the present. Who knows what she has in store for us in the future? As Linda has always done throughout her long career, her amazing book celebrates women's beauty.

—Felicia Rogawska Milewicz, Beauty Director, *Glamour* magazine

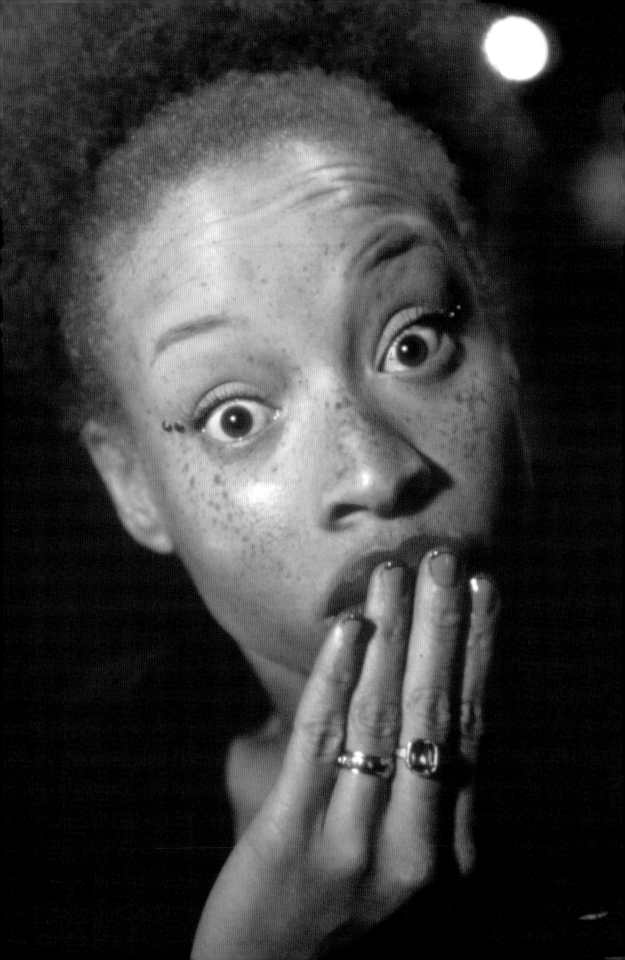

makeup as
self-discovery

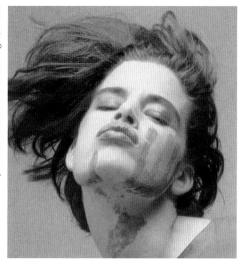

Photo by Steven Meisel for German Vogue, 1984.

I have always enjoyed makeup—it has brought excitement and fun into both my personal and professional life. But I also believe that makeup is a true art form: the practice of applying and wearing it involves vast expressive possibilities.

Many other makeup artists who have written beauty books or who give makeup lessons do so by reinforcing certain standards to which one should conform in order to look beautiful. *This book is not about standards.* It is, rather, a handbook of *techniques and approaches* that I have developed and refined over an incredible quarter-century career making up all different types of people from all different walks of life. The results of my experience are distilled in this book. In my work, I am constantly confronted by questions about beauty and makeup: The answers I have found throughout the various twists and turns in my career are here. My aim in *Makeup: The Art of Beauty* is not only to inspire you to try new techniques, but also to encourage your confidence to experiment with, enjoy, and use makeup as a personality-enhancing accessory. The tips and techniques I present in this book are those that I have used most in my life and work; they work as well in real life with real women as they do on the runway or on a photo shoot with models and actresses.

Yes, there are some rules, and applying makeup by following them will allow you to emphasize and enhance the beauty of your *features,* but once you experiment a bit with some of the different techniques in this book, you will also be able to accentuate your *personality* as well as your physical beauty. That may happen when you break some of those rules.

A model back stage at the 1996 Cynthia Rowley show in New York. She's wearing lilac cream eye shadow, violet eyeliner, violet lip color, and no base or concealer on her skin. I attached jewels near the end of her outer lash line with false-eyelash glue. *Photo by David Webber*

People always ask me to name the most beautiful woman I have ever made up. I find the question impossible to answer. Often, a beauty that strikes one immediately pales more quickly than a beauty that grows on you and takes time to be discovered. In the studio or behind the scenes at a show, many times a model would sit down to be made up and I would think, "Gosh, what is *she* doing here?" By the time I had finished doing her makeup, I had often totally changed mind and found her very beautiful, and not just because of the makeup! While working, I would "discover" her, so to speak, and by the time I had finished, I understood. Many models really were once ugly ducklings who transformed into swans—not because of plastic surgery—but because someone who could *see* the beauty in them took the pains to make them feel good and capture their spirit on camera. This doesn't happen overnight —I saw girls slowly grow more and more beautiful as they became more confident. Using makeup to express your sense of yourself also brings about such transformations. A woman who looks and feels good without makeup is beautiful; but playfully adding a dash of color and light or even transforming oneself totally and baffling the world can feel magical.

That's why I say that makeup has the power to bring fairy tales to life.

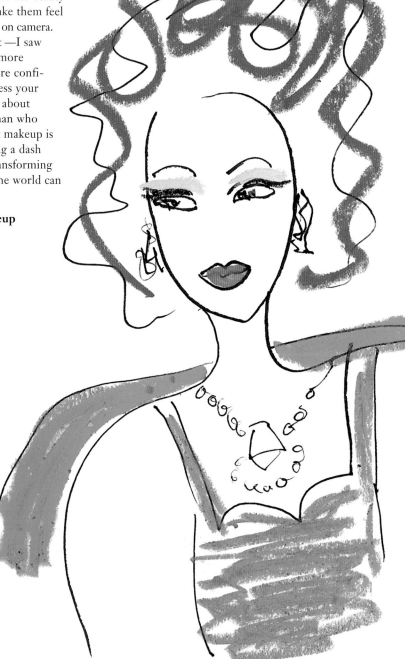

my early career Inspiration and Training

I grew up reading every fairy tale I could find, but none compared to the one I lived every day watching my mother apply her makeup.

The French cosmetic line Lancôme was my pale-skinned, redheaded mother's favorite. It seemed very exotic to me, a little girl from the north of England. She would do all the classic steps in the right order. First you applied the concealer, followed by foundation, face powder, eye makeup, blush, and finally, lipstick. That's how makeup was done then; it had to be *complete*. When I first became a makeup artist, I thought making a face into a blank canvas and reconstructing it with makeup was lots of fun. I still enjoy doing that, but it's not the only way or even necessarily the best way to make someone look fabulous. Different people have different lifestyles; makeup should reflect that. With a little knowledge of the effects that can be obtained with certain techniques and tools, you can express your personality and embark on a journey of self-discovery. When you apply particular products to your face they will in some way, however slight, highlight your features on their own and bring out your individuality.

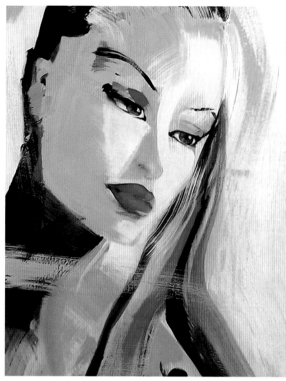

Prayer Hands, Linda Mason, 1999. Acrylic on canvas, 36 x 48 in (91.5 x 122 cm).

My awareness of light and its effect on surfaces and colors has always influenced me. Sunderland, my coal-mining, shipbuilding hometown in the north of England, seemed dark and drab to many, but by filling our house with windows, glass brick walls, and mirrors, my mother gave our home a beautiful, soft, embellishing light. She inspired me and encouraged me to travel and have fun. I was doing just that in Beirut and Lebanon, working as a sales representative for a perfume manufacturer, when a client suggested I contact Lancôme. I ended up training to be a makeup artist for the company that inspired me when I was a child.

I began my makeup training in Paris with Monsieur Ulysse, Lancôme's wonderful makeup artist, then traveled back to Beirut to work for Lancôme both selling and teaching makeup to the beautiful golden-green-eyed Lebanese women.

At the beginning of the '70s, I returned to Paris and changed my career for a while by becoming a model. I kept my makeup skills going by teaching at "Elle Club," where young women came to learn new beauty tricks. There, in 1975, I had the opportunity to watch another great makeup artist, Jacques Clement, and was also given my first chance to do makeup for a photo shoot by the French cosmetic company Isabelle Lancray. The photographer, Sammy Georges, was excellent, and the results of our work launched my career as a makeup artist.

When I was offered the chance to model in Japan for six weeks at the beginning of 1976, I seized the opportunity. The experience influenced me in many ways: The richness of the culture, the colorful kimonos, and the theater all gave me something to draw upon later. My love of red eyeliner is just one of the many Japanese influences on my work.

Upon returning to Paris, I was offered a position at Helena Rubinstein as their head makeup artist. I worked on magazine shoots and in-house shoots for public relations and advertising. I also trained the instructors of the store makeup artists, did seasonal color stories for magazines and the company, and did special promotions in different countries.

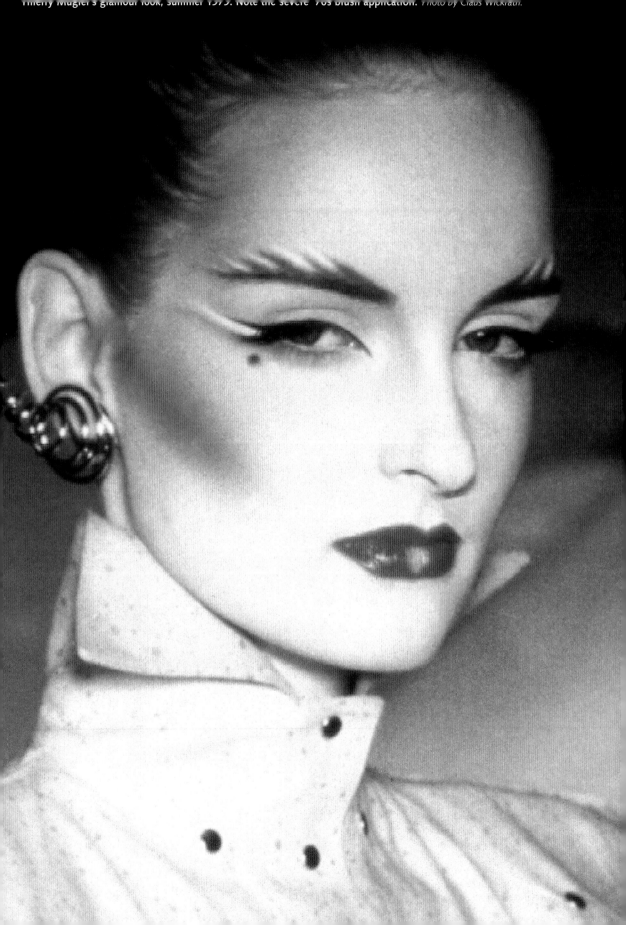

my **work** in the World of Fashion

One of my first assignments for Helena Rubinstein in the fall of 1976 was to do the prêt-à-porter fashion shows in Italy, and I continued to return to Italy to do the shows each season for another three years. Everything was incredibly well organized by the combined efforts of the Italian makeup artists and Monsieur Franco Savorelli, a wonderful public relations professional for the Italian branch of Helena Rubinstein (he worked on a freelance basis). The six to eight shows a day I was working became a blur, but two very different designers with whom I worked that first season left a lasting impression on me: Walter Albini, whose flair for color and innovative and extravagant designs inspired me to go wild with makeup, and Giorgio Armani, with his extremely flattering, beautifully cut suits for women, for whom I did a much more subdued, soft, classic pink look. The French fashion shows in 1976 were a different matter. There was an explosion of designer talent, but when

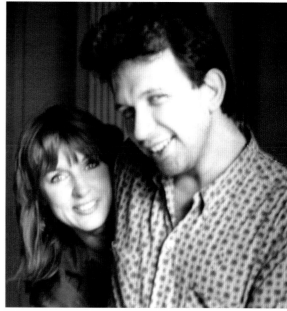

Linda Mason and Jean Paul Gaultier, 1979.

I was sent by the company to do the makeup, makeup artists were just expected to drop off the makeup and let the models do their thing. I sat in on a show at Jean Patou and noticed that there was a big difference between what the models were wearing on their faces and the clothes they wore on their bodies. Angelo Tarlazzi was the Patou designer at that time, and his clothes were very inspiring. I knew I had to get the models to change their makeup so that it would be more in harmony with the statement the designer was making. To my joy, I managed to actually do the makeup on each model and change her look. From then on, I was hooked on doing makeup for the shows. To prepare, I would go in and meet with the designer, and, depending on the designer, either make suggestions about colors and styles, or actually do a makeup on one of his or her assistants. I learned a lot, especially from Thierry Mugler, a total perfectionist who taught me lots of little details and why they were important, and who also showed me the enormous difference a tiny fraction in placement can make to makeup.

For my first Thierry Mugler show, the models were made up in a "degrade" of green, from the palest shades on the skin to a dark green Unibrow. I was feeling rather pleased with myself after having successfully completed some of the first makeup back stage when a large group of '70s star models—Jerry Hall, Pat Cleveland, etc.— arrived. They gasped in horror and swore I would come nowhere near their faces. Once they calmed down, I crept up on them and managed to make them conform slightly to the required "look."

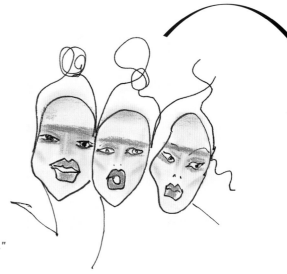

Evolutions in Style

Working with a designer over a number of seasons is important. It gives you the opportunity to evolve and grow together, as I was able to do with Jean Paul Gaultier, with whom I worked from 1978 until 1985. Jean Paul was the first designer on whose models I started doing individualized makeup, as opposed to one theme on all the models. His paper clothing and mechanical jewelry inspired me to break out of the mold of symmetrical, predictable makeup. Another initiating force in this breakthrough also came towards the end of the '70s. I did a group of dancers in Paris from the "Crazy Horse Salon" (a more erotic form of the "Moulin Rouge") for a photo shoot for American *Cosmopolitan* magazine. The star of the show never removed her makeup; she slept in it. Despite her protests, I removed her messy black makeup to begin afresh. She could not even look at herself in the mirror without her makeup on and became very emotional. She started crying, and I thought, "What am I trying to do tidying up her makeup?" She had looked absolutely gorgeous with her thick, black messy signature eye makeup. This expression of her individuality was what had made her into the star of the show. These experiences taught me the importance of understanding the personality of the person on whom you are applying makeup, and that perfection and the classical rules of makeup are not necessarily the best ways to accentuate a person's beauty, individuality, or to express a mood. As I've said, sometimes rules should be broken.

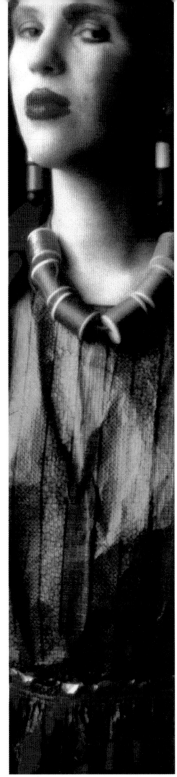

I thought Jean Paul Gaultier's paper clothes needed a different type of makeup, such as this freestyle look.
Model: Melody.

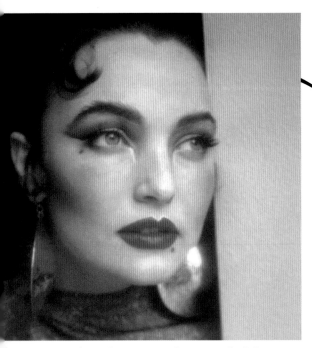

"Nina" with a softer, warmer glamourous look for a Thierry Mugler shoot, 1980. See page 14 for similar white detail in the upswept eye makeup.

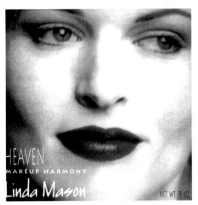

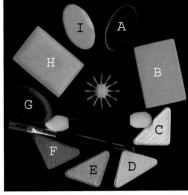

Heaven makeup kit. This is part of my "Harmonies" makeup line based on mixing and layering color within certain color palettes. Colors can be mixed or layered to create different looks ranging from soft and transparent to dramatic and sophisticated.

During this same time, in the late '70s, I searched out designers such as Issey Miyake whose clothes I loved, then persuaded them they needed me. Initially, I had teams of makeup artists assisting me in Milan, but when I worked in Paris, I would prepare diagrams and kits of color for each of the models and do the makeup on some of the girls really early so that as the others were arriving, they could see the uniform style that was required.

Doing the shows made me realize that when you decide to make a style change, whether it be a dramatic new dress or just a slight change in your hair, you should take the opportunity to rethink your makeup. Put on your new dress before applying your makeup, or begin your makeup by first applying your newest product, then adapt the rest of your makeup to that new color.

When I did not have assistants, I would make a drawing and a kit of the colors and products I wanted the models to use, then make sure I spent a few minutes with each of them, adjusting their makeup to make sure it conformed to the "makeup design" the fashion designer and I had agreed upon. To this day, I love putting together palettes of color to enable a woman to transform herself the way I transformed the models then: by mixing and layering color. This method of working inspired my color kits—"Moodkits" in 1987, "Harmonies" in 1995, "Melodies" in 1998, and "Mini Masterpieces" in 2000.

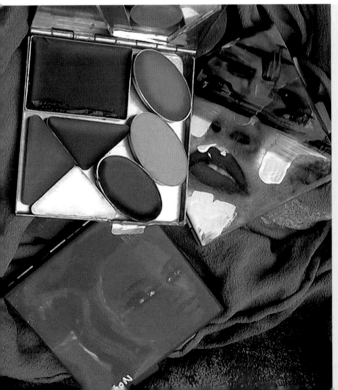

Mini Masterpiece Color Kit: All Lips

You can create any lip color you like by mixing these colors. Clockwise from top left:

Tinted black gloss will make any lip color glossier and creamier. It will also slightly deepen either your natural lip tone or another lip color.

Orange can be used alone or with another color to make it more warm and orange.

Nude will lighten other colors. For a soft look, use it with gloss.

Brown will deepen other colors and make them more muted. To define lips, outline them with brown and softly blend around the edges.

Pearl makes other colors lighter and pearlier.

Red Hot mixed with orange makes a nice orange-red shade.

Ruby makes darker colors cooler and makes lighter colors a bit cooler/bluer by adding a touch of pink.

Asian Influences

At the end of the '70s, I spent a few months in Japan—this time as a makeup artist. I started doing my own photography and experimenting with a set of traditional makeup that the Japanese cosmetics company Shiseido had given me as a gift. It was liberating to do my own photography, and I gained a greater understanding of a photographer's needs, such as that for 100 percent of the makeup artist's attention.

While in Japan, I did the makeup for quite a few designer shows, and I was extremely impressed by Yohji Yamamoto's designs. However, it was a designer for whose show I did not work who impressed me the most: Rei Kawakubo. I had always felt that no designer had yet created modern clothing that accentuated the beauty of Japanese women as the traditional kimono did. When I saw Rei's clothing, I was very excited—her clothes challenged the accepted fashion conventions and were nothing like Japanese clothing, yet they somehow managed to enhance the spirit and shape of the Japanese woman as beautifully as a kimono did.

You can imagine my excitement when Rei's stylist Mako asked me to do Rei's first show in Paris in the fall of 1981. Even before I went to meet her, I knew that a traditional makeup would not be right for her innovative, deconstructed clothing. I was told Rei wanted "makeup," but didn't like "makeup," which I understood to mean that she disliked "traditional" makeup. Rei suggested two circles of rouge in the center of the cheeks. I knew that to create the right effect, the traditional style of makeup should be deconstructed,

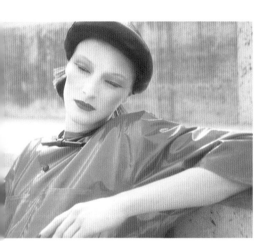

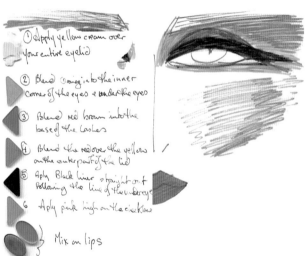

Designer Anne Marie Beretta always gave me a strong direction for her makeup, as seen in her detailed notebook sketch (right) and in the resulting realized makeup in the photo (left). *Illustration by Anne Marie Beretta.*

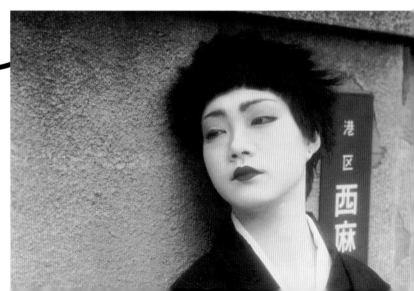

Yoshimi with wig, 1979. I was experimenting with traditional Japanese stage makeup given to me by Shisheido, using it to create a more modern look. *Hair by Tetsu Tamurayama of MOD'S Hair Japan.*

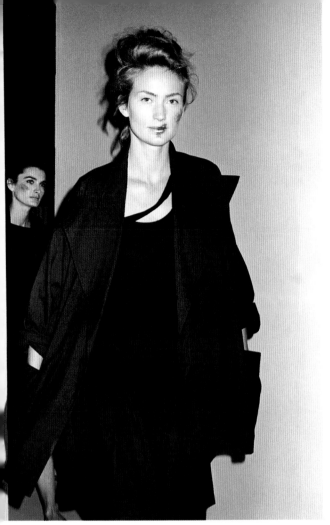

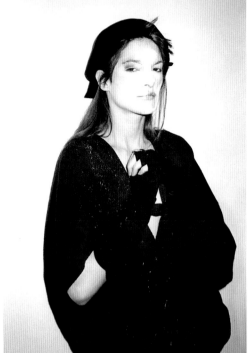

ABOVE **Lynn back stage at the Fall Comme Des Garçons show in March of 1982. Pushing the boundaries of makeup to complement Rei Kawakubo's designs.**

LEFT **Anna modeling the Spring 1983 Comme Des Garçons collection in Paris in October, 1982. Lipstick pressed onto the lips, and cream blushes pressed onto the cheeks.** *Both photos by Roxanne Lowit*

therefore it was essential to eliminate base, concealer, and mascara (three components of makeup models never did a show without). Most of the models had great skin with slight dark circles under their eyes, but they were all insecure and believed they needed it. Now we are used to seeing nude faces, but at the beginning of the '80s, we had not yet exited from the excesses of the disco '70s. With Rei's help, at the rehearsal the night before the show, we succeeded in getting most of the girls to remove their base, and I applied two unblended rounds of blush to their cheeks, and then watched the rehearsal. That night, I saw that there was something more that needed to be done. The following morning, I went very early to the show and spoke to Rei about adding splashes of bright blue and green cream shadow asymmetrically to certain girls' eyelids. We tried it out, and Rei cautiously accepted using it on certain girls. It was a bit difficult to get the girls themselves to realize that they could still look attractive. But once the show started, the reaction and excitement from the models was so great, they all wanted color, and everything went incredibly well. The models really got the whole feeling of the show. They *understood* it!

For her fall collection (shown in the spring of 1982), Rei requested a monochromatic earth-toned makeup in the same vein as the previous season. I wanted to break up the earth tones with an almost imperceptible touch of a light, bright, cool blue, but I couldn't really explain why. After the show, when journalists kept coming up to congratulate me on my great "battered woman" look, I regretted not having stuck to my guns about the addition of color. If you push the boundaries, you are vulnerable to other people's interpretations of your experiments, but what was most important was that the makeup complimented Rei's designs. Roxanne Lowit, the first photographer to work back stage at the Paris prêt-à-porter, captured this.

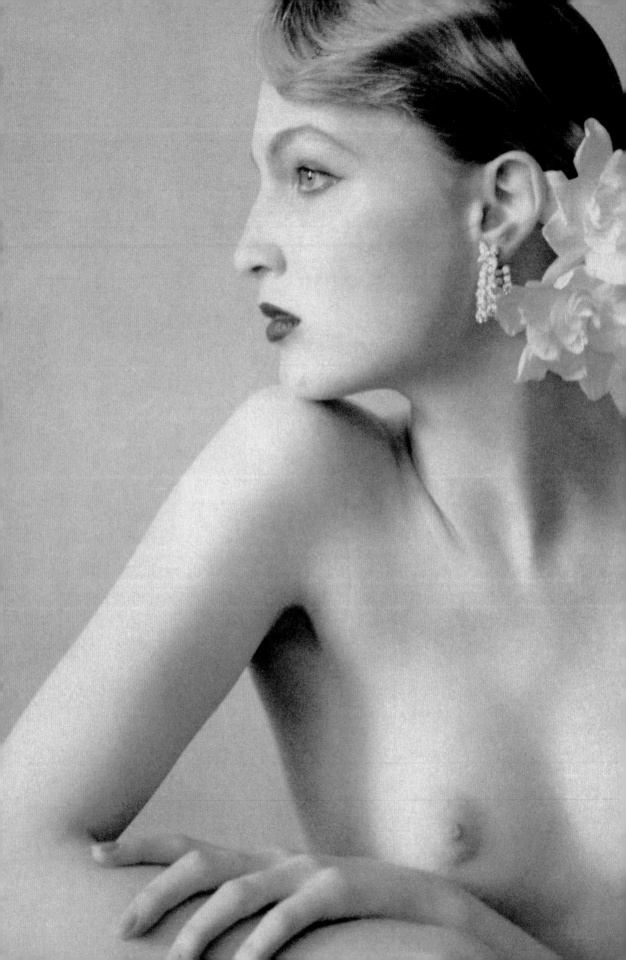

american style

Always on the quest for a new adventure, I moved to the States. The first American designer with whom I worked was Stephen Sprouse, whose neon, glow-in-the-dark suits and graffiti mini-skirts were incredibly fun and inspiring. Stephen loved dark, smudgy black eyes with pale lips. Spurred on by the photographer Stephen Meisel, with whom I frequently worked, I gave this throwback look from the '60s a modern approach, applying the black asymmetrically in a strong, sloppy manner with a paintbrush. New to New York and inspired by the street art I was seeing, I was doing a lot of "graffiti" on the face, so for Sprouse's second show, he chose the words he wanted, and I wrote them in inverted "graffiti" on the models' faces, again with a dark, smoky eye.

Debbie Harry with a signature smoky eye that looks as good today as it did in 1982.
Photo by Guzman. Art Direction: Stephen Sprouse. Hair: Christian.

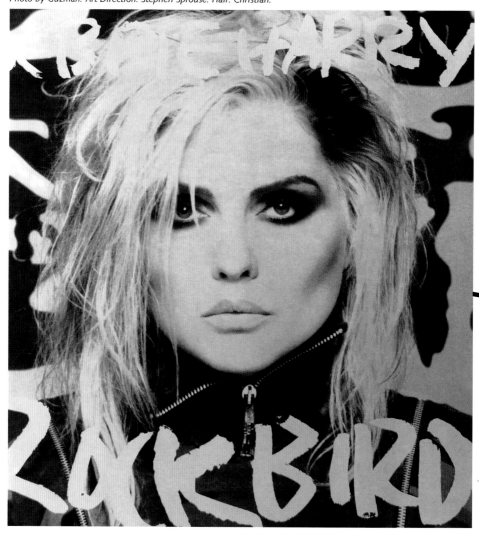

OPPOSITE PAGE **Model Rebecca's complexion is pale, translucent, and extremely luminous. This type of skin can be easily dulled by a base or powder. It may only need a thin film of white base, if any. I applied turquoise shadow to her lids and a thin line of red eyeliner.** *Photo by Sheila Metzner, 1985. Hair by Gerard Bollei.*

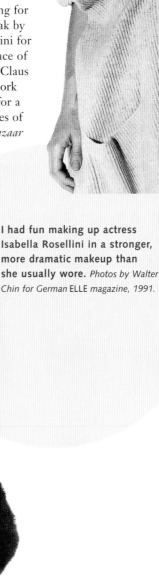

New York, New York

Diametrically different styles existed side by side in fashion and makeup in the '80s, so I found myself working for more traditional U.S. designers, such as Perry Ellis and Lois D'Ell Olio of Anne Klein. Then, in 1987, British Designer of the Year John Galliano came to New York; after working with him there, I traveled to London to do his shows and his advertising with the photographer Javier Vallhonrat. John is a treasure and an inspiration. No matter what kind of pressure he's under, he remains constantly upbeat and fun, and he knows how to make people comfortable enough to give their best.

The photographers living in New York whom I had worked with in Paris were very faithful to their makeup artists in New York, and I didn't find getting work so easy upon my arrival. I had, however, met the beauty editor of *Mademoiselle* magazine, Felicia Milewicz, on a previous visit to New York. She booked me to work for *Mademoiselle* and spoke to the fashion photographer Deborah Turbeville, with whom I had loved working for Italian *Vogue* in Paris. Deborah then gave me a break by booking me for a photo shoot with Isabella Rossellini for American *Vogue* magazine, which stepped up the pace of my career. Before leaving Paris, the photographer Claus Wickrath gave me the opportunity to do creative work splashing color on models using products like jam for a photography show he was preparing. With the slides of this show, I tried to persuade *Vogue* and *Harper's Bazaar* to do something similar.

I had fun making up actress Isabella Rosellini in a stronger, more dramatic makeup than she usually wore. *Photos by Walter Chin for German ELLE magazine, 1991.*

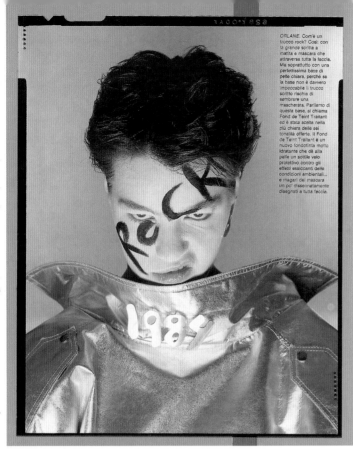

ORLANE. Com'è un trucco rock? Così: con la grande scritta a matita e mascara che attraversa tutta la faccia. Ma soprattutto con una perfettissima base di pelle chiara, perché se la base non è davvero impeccabile il trucco scritto rischia di sembrare una mascherata. Parliamo di questa base, si chiama Fond de Teint Traitant ed è stata scelta nella più chiara delle sei tonalità offerte. Il Fond de Teint Traitant è un nuovo fondotinta molto idratante che dà alla pelle un sottile velo protettivo contro gli effetti essiccanti delle condizioni ambientali... e magari dei mascara un po' dissonatamente disegnati a tutta faccia.

Facial graffiti for a beauty shoot with Steven Meisel and Stephen Sprouse.

The photo below was for a fashion-shoot with designer John Galliano's clothes. It has a '20s or '30s feel. The eyebrows are widely spaced: I drew a thin, descending black line with an eyebrow pencil approximately one quarter of an inch after the beginning of the natural eyebrows and above the natural brow line. The lip makeup was inspired by the style popular in the '20s of accentuating the Cupid's bow.

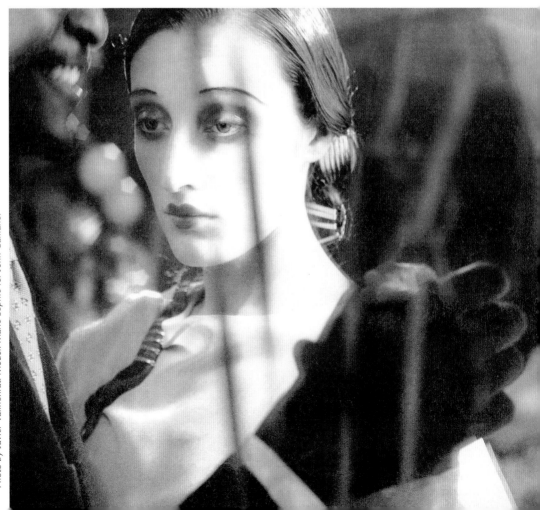

Breaking in

Carlotta Jacobsen, then beauty director of American *Harper's Bazaar*, succeeded (although it took her six months) in having an article on breaking the rules in makeup published. After that article came out, and after the publication of the other work I was doing at that time with Steven Meisel, work started flowing in. Magazines such as Italian *Vogue* and German *Stern* gave me free rein. The stronger features of the models that were popular in the '80s lent themselves to asymmetrical, unusual makeup. Often, inspired by the movement of the models and the effects of the lighting, I applied makeup more on the set while the shoot was in progress instead of making up the model in the changing room.

I was fortunate enough to have always worked on interesting advertising campaigns and commercials in Paris, and I continued to do so in New York and Europe. Projects such as the Alexon campaign with Richard Avedon and Iman, inspired by African makeup, and the German Jewelry campaign for Neissing with the photographer Helmut Hoffmann enabled me to express myself with color. They were also the shoots that inspired me to paint.

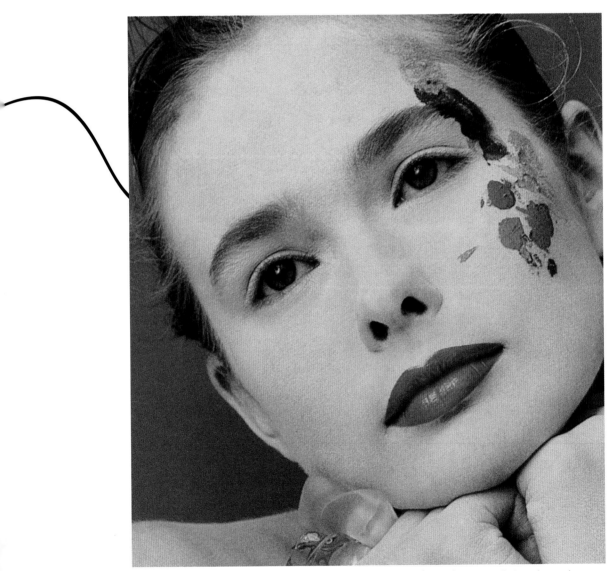

White Kabuki makeup made modern with an asymmetrical, freestyle approach to color and luscious, classic lips. *Photo by Art Kane for* Harper's Bazaar, 1983.

Helmut Hoffmann booked me on advertising campaigns for Neissing jewellery over a number of seasons. Helmut focused small beams of light onto the jewelry to accentuate it and told me to be equally creative with the model's makeup.
Photo by Helmut Hoffmann. Model: Anneliese. Art Direction: Martina Ibbels. Hair: Charles Olivier.

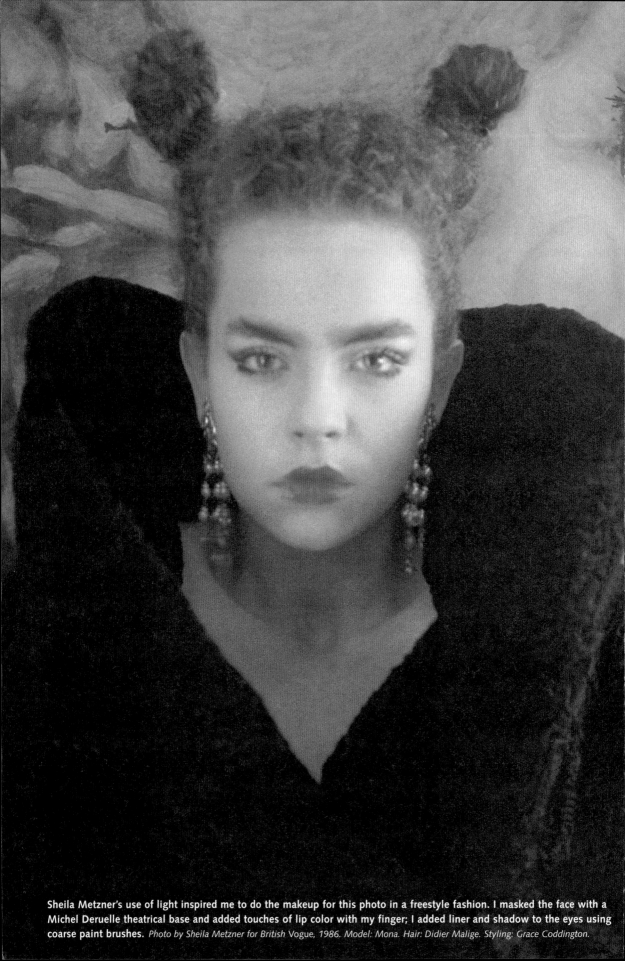

Sheila Metzner's use of light inspired me to do the makeup for this photo in a freestyle fashion. I masked the face with a Michel Deruelle theatrical base and added touches of lip color with my finger; I added liner and shadow to the eyes using coarse paint brushes. *Photo by Sheila Metzner for British* Vogue, *1986. Model: Mona. Hair: Didier Malige. Styling: Grace Coddington.*

I was never bored, even working on catalogue shoots for Bergdorf Goodman or more traditional advertising jobs for companies such as Revlon and Almay. The photographers I worked with were real pros and were full of love and enthusiasm for their work, even though some had been in the business for many years.

For a makeup artist, each day is a new adventure. I traveled back and forth to Europe and elsewhere and ventured to exotic locations such as the Seychelles and the Canary Islands (with my baby daughter Daisy now in tow) with photographers such as Hans Feurer and Matthew Rolston. I worked with many great beauties (who also happened to be budding starlets) such as Brooke Shields, Uma Thurman, and Famke Janssen. Work in the fashion industry sounds glamorous and fun; it is. It sounds superficial; it is. Another frequently heard notion is that models are airheads: They are most certainly not. They are beautiful and intelligent, not always easy to work with, but I cannot help but respect and admire even those with whom I have had difficulties. Fashion is a tough industry. If models are weak, they will not survive.

In 1990, the Japanese photographer Seiichi Tanaka approached the painter Marc Kostabi and me and asked if we would work together on a book with him. Both Marc and I had met Mr. Tanaka when we participated in one of his earlier book projects. We each brought a different sensibility to the project, which ended up being a book published in Japan called *Tanaka Mason Kostabi.* It was a great, very spontaneous experience. The book had no real concept, which meant we could be totally intuitive with the blending of our talents. One of us would have an idea or feeling, we might or might not talk about it, or we might just go off and start working. The celebrity or friend we were working on might also participate, and often their simple refusal to wear makeup took the project in an unexpected direction. People like to put things in boxes and label them: "You did the makeup and he did the painting." In reality, it wasn't that simple. That book, like my makeup store, is something people don't understand right away; it makes them think and wonder a bit.

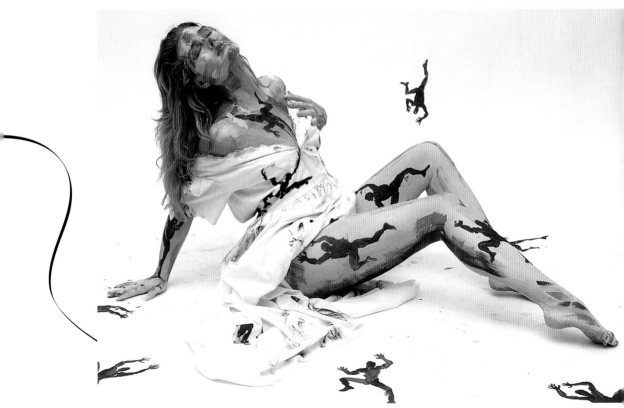

I asked Brooke Shields to be photographed for a book project I did with Seiichi Tanaka and Mark Kostabi. I loved working with Brooke and felt the book would give me the perfect opportunity to tap into her more provocative side. *Photo by Tanaka/Mason/Kostabi, 1990.*

Trends and the Times

The freedom people experienced in the '80s became more confined in the '90s. The fashion business became more serious. In the '80s, the models worked hard. They had a lusty love of life, had fun, went on to be artists, have creative careers, go back to college, or marry and have families. They all (even the difficult ones) enjoyed the experimental process of makeup. In the early to mid '90s, glamour—stylish makeup accentuating features in a conventional manner—returned with a vengeance. Makeup was tailored: matte and brown. Models became extremely image-conscious and career-oriented: this was the era of the "celebrity model," with Cindy Crawford, Naomi Campbell, Linda Evangelista, and Claudia Schiffer dominating the fashion pages. In the middle of the decade, Kate Moss came along and broke the mold with her carefree attitude and her fresh beauty, and as the decade progressed, a spirit of adventure returned.

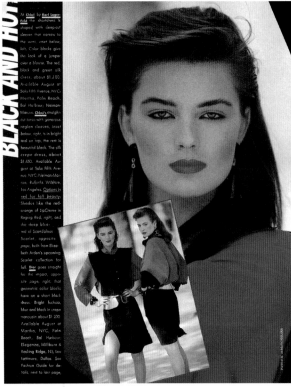

Paulina Poriskova, the hot new model in Paris, had just turned fifteen when Patrick did this photo for American *Harper's Bazaar.* Photo by Patrick Demarchelier, 1982.

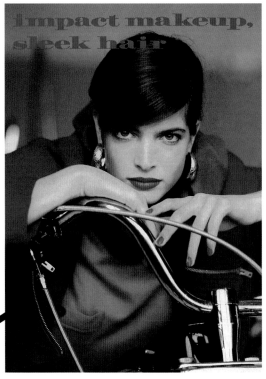

Model Stephanie Seymour on location in New York.
Photo by Arthur Elgort/ Mademoiselle, © Condé Nast Publications Inc.

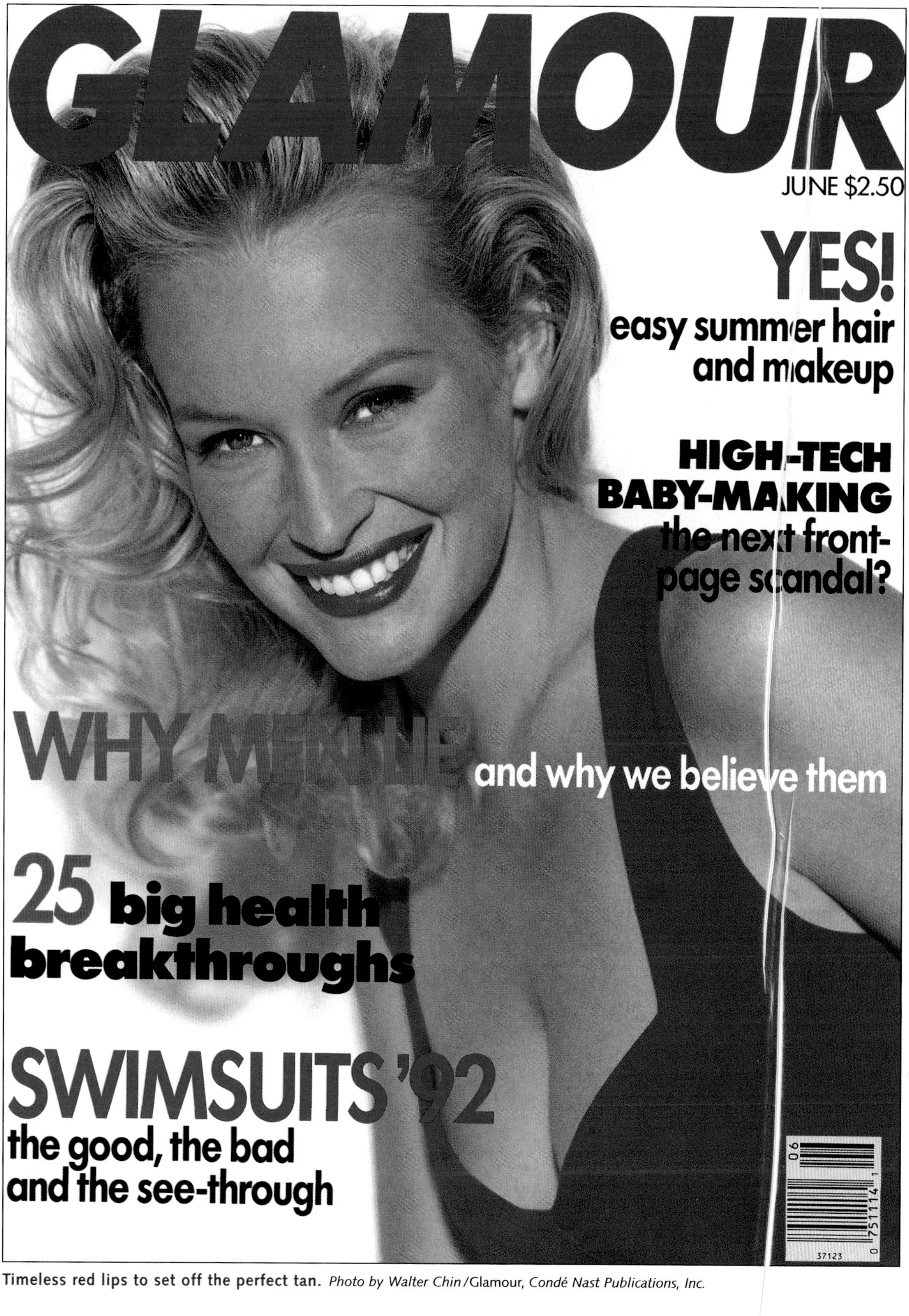

GLAMOUR

JUNE $2.50

YES!
easy summer hair and makeup

HIGH-TECH BABY-MAKING
the next front-page scandal?

WHY ME BLIEVE

and why we believe them

25 big health breakthroughs

SWIMSUITS '92
the good, the bad and the see-through

Timeless red lips to set off the perfect tan. *Photo by Walter Chin /Glamour, Condé Nast Publications, Inc.*

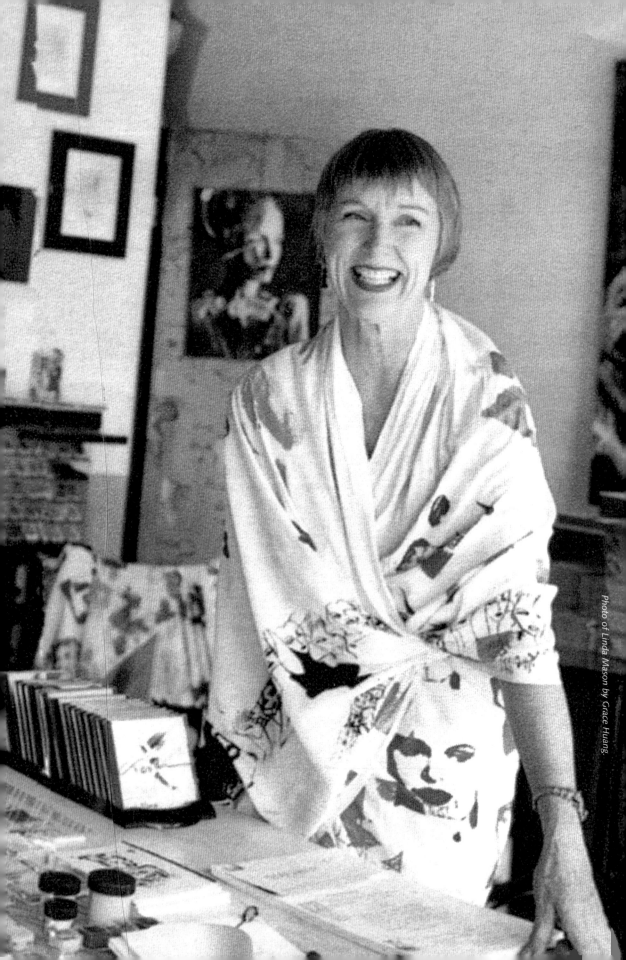

my makeup and my store

I started my cosmetic company, Linda Mason Elements, in 1987 and launched it at Henri Bendel, Barney's, then Nordstroms in California and Harrods of London in 1988. As a single mother eagerly attacking the cosmetic industry on every front, I soon found I had to work twice as hard to survive. I wasn't focused; my attention was spread too thin. To save my sanity, I pulled back and kept my products only in Barney's New York until 1992.

From 1992 to 1998, the year I opened my own shop, I kept my creative spirit fueled with my artwork and painting. I also launched a few cosmetic products, including the Daisy M. product line (inspired by and created with my daughter Daisy) in 1996. Also around this time, I began working on a wonderful group of actresses and actors here in New York, including Camryn Manheim, Cameron Diaz, Claire Danes, Elizabeth Berkly, Jeff Goldblum, and Don Henley.

When the events of my life led me to become a makeup artist in 1975, I could not believe my luck. Finally I had found the missing link: Work that wasn't work, but something about which I was so passionate, it was just like an extension of me. To pass along this experience of fulfillment, in 1998, in a small space with great light in SoHo in New York City, I opened my studio/boutique "The Art of Beauty by Linda Mason." It is a place where people—women and men—can come and be inspired by color and also get a deeper understanding of the fact that makeup is not just something you mask on to look respectable or change your features, but a beautiful part of life and an art form. I wrote this book for the same reason I opened my store: I want people to see that makeup can be a means of self-discovery. I hope the following chapters will help bring you the same spirit of enjoyment and creativity I have found in my work.

Linda Mason in her SoHo, New York studio.

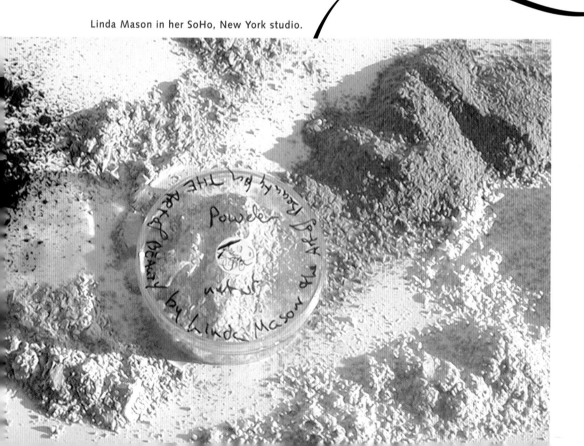

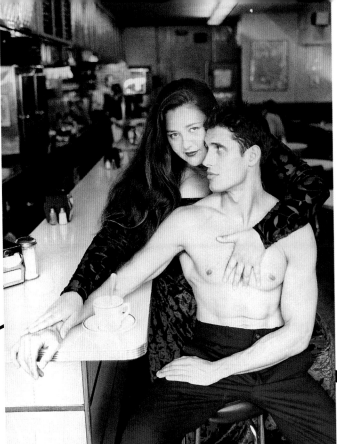

This was the first time I had worked with Camryn Manheim, and I had a great time transforming her face and getting to know her. Her favorite look is the strong, smoky eye. *Photo by Gerhard Yurkovic for MODE Magazine, 1998.*

A brown lip color makes this turquoise eye color look more elegant on model **Rachel Hunter.** *Photo by Jacques Malignon.*

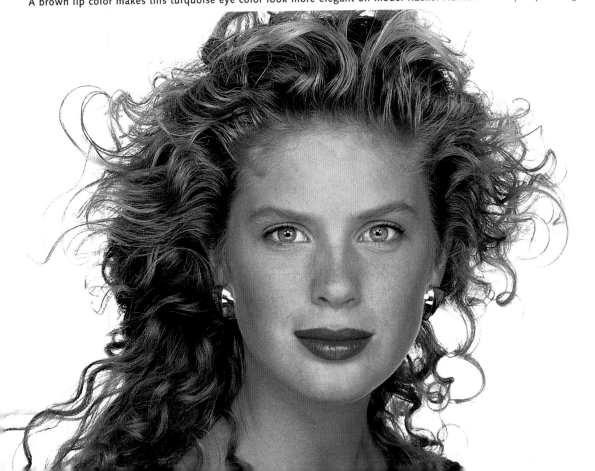

about this book

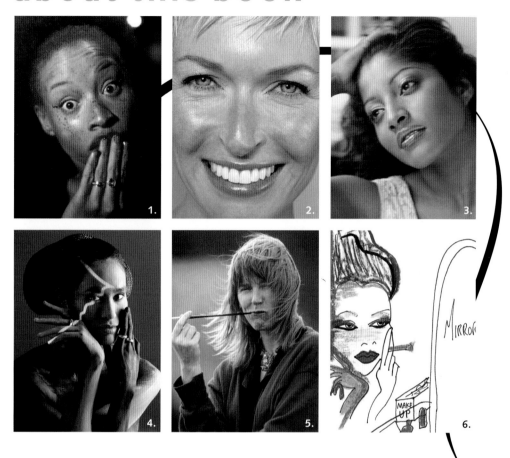

1. 2. 3. 4. 5. 6.

Chapter 1: "Makeup as Self-Discovery" explains my philosophy on makeup and beauty and outlines my inspiration, training, and career as a makeup artist.

Chapter 2: "Basics" introduces you to simple makeup techniques and tools. It helps you discover how you can use one technique to highlight your features, and how a combination of techniques can also complement your personality.

Chapter 3: "Glamourizing Techniques" will take you through the makeup styles popular throughout the 20th century. This chapter shows you how classic makeup techniques and styles from the past have been translated in contemporary styles, and it also shows you how to create such high-glamour, dramatic looks on yourself or others.

Chapter 4: "Freestyle" explains the freestyle techniques and tools that enable you to break out of the mold and experiment with makeup.

Chapter 5: "Professional Makeup" and **Chapter 6: "Becoming a Makeup Artist"** address all the questions I am routinely asked, not just by people wanting to become makeup artists, but also by those curious about the fashion industry and about just what being a makeup artist entails.

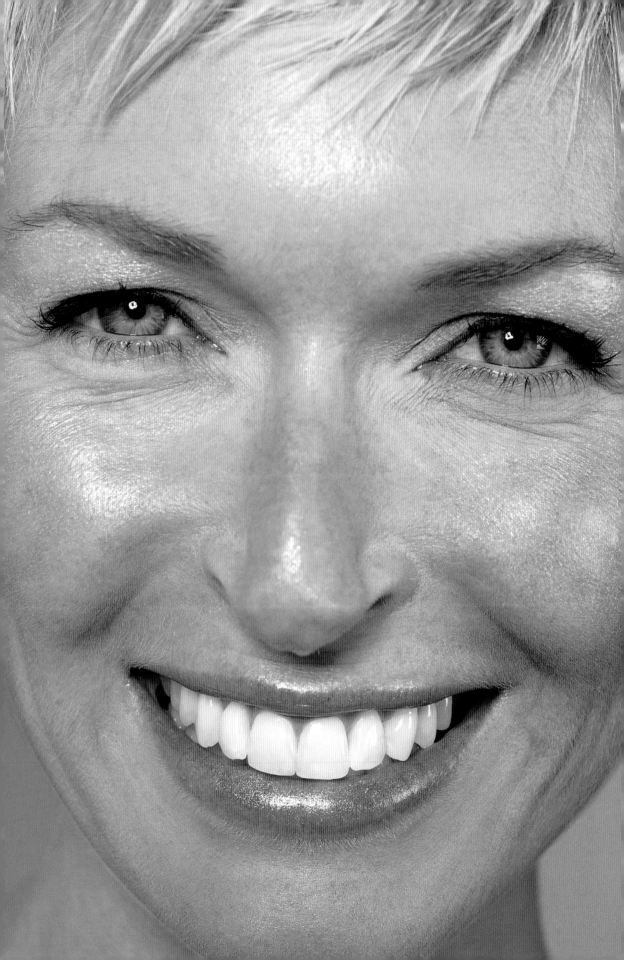

basics

Each face is a canvas, but not a blank one. Each face has features that make it unique. The simple, easy techniques that I call "the basics" gently enhance features by either accentuating them or altering their appearance slightly. Changing the positioning of a makeup product by a fraction of an inch can totally change its effect.

Not only does your face have its own color, texture, shape, and "personality," makeup itself comes in a daunting range of colors, textures, forms, and packages. So, with the aim of helping you with these basic choices, this chapter also encompasses the tools and products I have used the most throughout my career—the items I consider essential as both a makeup artist and a woman.

As far as color goes, there are a few basic rules, but I often find myself breaking them. Even though I have built my reputation on my use of color, I have had great difficulty trying to distill that expertise into simple guidelines. In fact, I almost excluded the subject from the "Basics" chapter—I feel strongly about a person being able to discover himself or herself through color. Your personality, mood, and sense of fashion will dictate many of your choices. I finally decided to just explain how *I* approach color—I hope I can help you achieve a level of knowledge and comfort that will enable you to develop your own approach.

For this fresh-faced look, the skin was warmed with a lightweight, water-based base applied very sparingly with a damp sponge. Concealer was applied under the eyes and around the nose and powdered for more staying power, and a warm, earthy shade of cream blush was blended over the cheekbones. A light, slightly pearlized shadow was applied over the entire eyelid, and brown liner was applied to the base of the upper lashes with black mascara. The brows were lightly penciled in with a taupe pencil. Slightly pearlized lip gloss was applied to the lips. *Photo by Bruno Gaget for* Good Housekeeping *magazine, 2001.*

skin Base, Concealer, and Powder

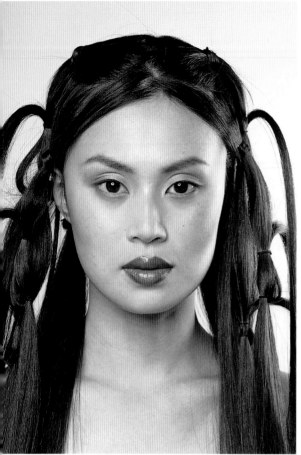

Not all of us are blessed with great skin; however, cosmetics companies are now producing bases of such superior quality that even problem skin can look great. Indeed, choosing a base (or deciding whether or not to use one) is the most important and perhaps the most difficult aspect of doing makeup. If you have problem skin but are caring for it properly, most bases will go on smoothly, and the texture of the base you use (cream or liquid) will just be a matter of personal preference. If you are not taking good care of your skin, then any base will have a tendency to sit on top of it, and you will always look more made up than someone who has soft, supple, well-cared-for skin. "Well cared for" means skin that is cleansed and moisturized, morning and night, even if you are only in your early teens. If I have misjudged someone's skin and the base does not go on as well as I expected, I will recleanse the face to remove the base immediately, then massage the skin with almond oil, which is light, highly absorbable, and which acts to stimulate and revitalize the skin. Keep the following factors in mind when deciding on the texture of your base.

Bruno Gaget (both photos this page).
Hair (both photos): Mayumi for
John Sahag.

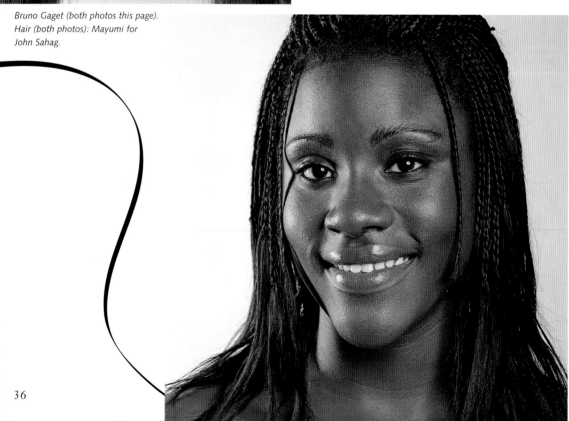

Base Textures: Cream vs. Liquid

The texture of a base will determine its finished effect on your skin, and although there are some cream bases with a light consistency, as a rule, a cream base gives a more matte coverage and a more sophisticated finish than a liquid base. Some women have skin that will soak up a liquid base so that it just disappears. Others have extremely uneven skin tone that benefits from the extra overall coverage of a cream base. Certain very oily complexions are actually best suited for a cream base because it blends well with the oils of the skin and gives a smooth finish. Some liquid bases give moderate to heavy coverage, but for a more fresh-faced look, either a lightweight, liquid base or just well-blended concealer applied to imperfections and under-eye circles is the best choice.

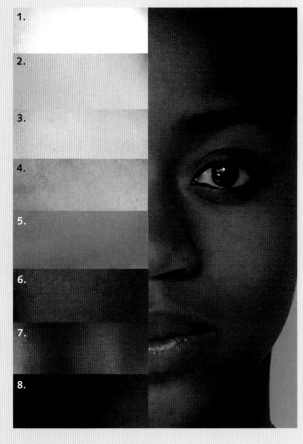

Check these skin tone "swatches" against the skin of your inner forearm and find the closest match.

1. Light ivory skin tone
2. Light skin, medium to pink undertone
3. Neutral light beige
4. Light olive skin
5. Warm, medium -toned skin
6. Olive skin
7. Brown to dark brown skin, red undertone
8. Blue-black skin tone

The population of the United States represents a wide range of skin tones. I use the bases pictured below most frequently. These base colors correspond to the skin tones in the photo to the left. If (and only if) your skin tone is one of the first three, and you would like to look more tan, use a base two to three shades darker than the one that matches your natural skin tone.

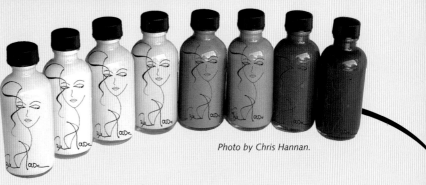

Photo by Chris Hannan.

Generally, I like liquid bases that are light-weight and water-based. The differences among products such as base, concealer, and powder are very subtle, and you can only see whether or not they enhance your skin when you actually apply them. If you are planning on wearing all three of these products together, then you should test all of them together. You don't need to apply them to your face to do so—just try them on the skin on the inside of your wrist or forearm. Try more than one color at once so you can compare and thereby make the best choice. Because it is in a protected area, the skin on your inner wrist or forearm is the best representation of your true skin tone and thus the best place to immediately see the hue and intensity of a base and its effect on your skin. Look at the color in daylight if possible.

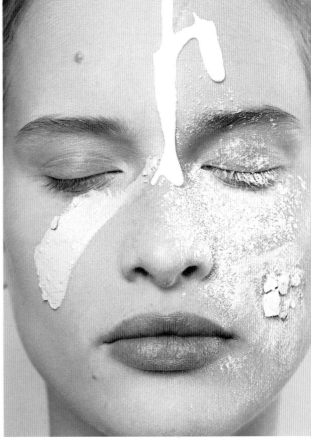

Clockwise from left: cream base, liquid base, loose powder, compact powder. *Photo by Bruno Gaget.*

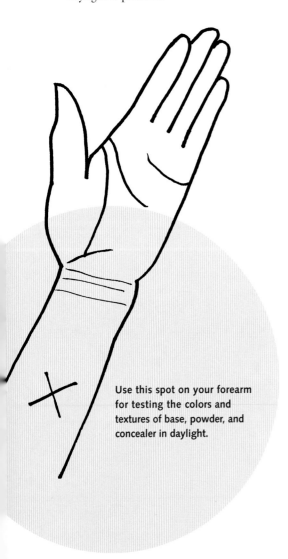

Use this spot on your forearm for testing the colors and textures of base, powder, and concealer in daylight.

If you want to match your base to your skin tone perfectly, the base's hue and depth of color should be the same as that of the skin of your inner forearm and should blend there imperceptibly. A fine liquid base will brighten the skin slightly; a heavier base will even out imperfections or patchiness.

However, you may want to enhance or alter your skin tone if you have a tanned body or wish to add warmth to your face. Some women prefer a warmer look, and changing your location can necessitate a change in the color of your base. If you are a New Yorker moving to Florida, for example, where the weather and the colors are sunnier and lighter, you may need a warmer foundation shade. When choosing a darker base, make sure you chose one the same hue as your skin tone; if you tend to use a lightweight base, just choose one about three shades deeper than the one that matches your skin tone most closely. When applying a dot of the base to the inner arm area, ask yourself, "Does this base make my skin duller?" If it does, it either contains a lot of gray or is the wrong hue and is therefore an unsuitable choice.

Concealer

Slight dark circles can be sexy, but if the circles are heavy or if you have close-set eyes, you should probably use concealer. In most cases, you should aim for a concealer in the same hue as your base, but slightly lighter. If you have difficulty finding something with the same undertone, choose a concealer a few shades lighter than your skin and mix it with your base. This method will not work, however, for someone whose skin is lighter around the eyes, either naturally or because they are often outdoors in sunny weather wearing glasses. If that is true for you, you will need to slightly deepen the color of the skin around your eyes. Even if you don't have dark circles, adding coverage to and lightening the area under the eye is desirable for evening makeup because you will, ideally, be getting a lot more close-up attention. You can dot on your concealer, and then blend it with your fingertips, but application and blending will be easier if you use a concealer brush first and then finish blending with your fingertip using a dabbing motion. After you apply base (if you are wearing any), apply concealer with a concealer brush to any blemishes and to the upper and lower inner corners of the eyes. The effect of this is three-fold: to cover any dark circles, to minimize the appearance of close-set eyes, and to help bring out deep-set eyes.

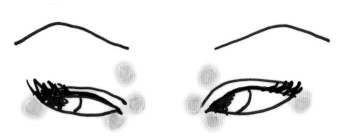

Apply concealer to the inner corners of the eyes and the under-eye area. Using concealer to slightly lighten the area just below the outer corners of the eyes will provide extra coverage in this area, which is often redder. Doing so will also give the face a little "lift."

Tools for the skin

Base, concealer and blush can all be applied with your fingertips, but you will get more precision using the correct tools or even using a mixture of the tools and your fingertips.

1. A concealer brush should be flat and have synthetic hairs; this is the best type of brush for applying creams.

2. A large, solid sponge used damp to apply your base can be washed frequently and will last.

3. A larger-headed, firm eyeshadow brush with natural hair should be kept clean. Use it to apply powder over concealer in the smaller areas of the face.

4. A powder puff made of cotton works well for applying powder to the larger areas of the face. Press the powder into the base to make the makeup last longer.

5. Sweep a clean, natural-haired blusher brush over the finished, powdered face to remove any extra powder.

6. An even larger brush with natural hair will remove any extra powder.

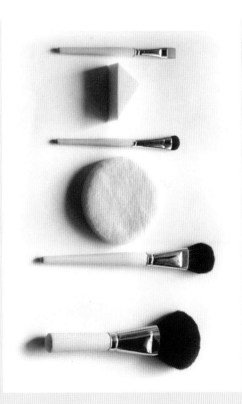

39

Powder

There are numerous varieties of powder and most have a certain amount of shine. A good matte translucent or transparent powder is very difficult to find. This is a powder that either lightens and brightens your base by a fraction, giving it a slight lift, or that does not alter the color of your base at all. Many so-called translucent powders can change the base dramatically. The main purpose of this powder is to give a matte finish to areas of the face in which you do not want shine, such as around the nose, the chin, and the forehead. Your nose will also look less prominent if you apply a matte powder to it rather than leaving it shiny. Powders in general should be pressed on the skin with a powder puff or a firm brush rather than fluffed on loosely; after all, their purpose is to make the makeup more matte and long-lasting. If you have applied too much powder, fluff off the excess with a larger brush. Today, compact powders tend to be lightweight, and loose powders often tend to be heavier. Shiny opalescent powders are wonderful for people with great skin and well-balanced, perfect features. If you do not have these but want to dust on a little shine, just dust it over certain parts of your face such as your cheekbones and put a little on your neck and body.

Many women make mistakes when choosing their powder. You should test it, too, on clean skin in daylight on your inner arm and then with the concealer and base with which you will be combining it. If the area becomes darker and duller, you know you have the wrong powder. If you have an exceptionally pale skin, as many redheads do, even translucent powders can dull your skin unless you first apply a light dusting of a white powder.

For darker-skinned women, a powder with the same hue as your underlying skin tone but with a stronger pigment is best. Apply a little translucent powder on the under-eye area and around the nose and chin before applying these more pigmented powders, as they can sometimes cause a deepening of the skin tone in those areas.

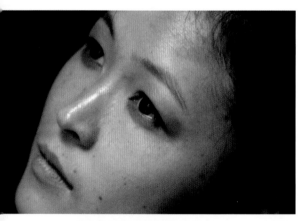

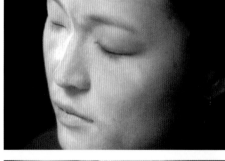

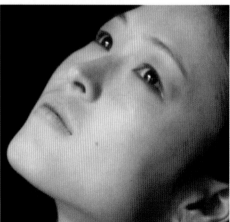

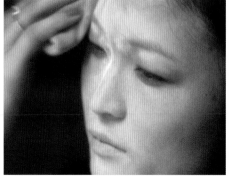

CLOCKWISE FROM TOP LEFT **For a well-powdered, matte face, start with moist skin. Distribute loose powder over the base. The pressing movement of the hand holding the cotton powder puff fixes the makeup and produces a matte, even finish.**

Using Base, Concealer, and Powder

A fresh-faced look

Step 1 For a fresh-faced look, dot the concealer under the eyes, on the imperfections, and softly pat to blend.

Step 2 Blend the concealer under the eyes and on blemishes.

Step 3 Apply powder over the parts of the face where there is concealer. Even when going for a creamy unpowdered look, I recommend powdering over the areas that have concealer with a small powder brush or large clean eye-shadow brush, to make sure it stays put and lasts a long time.

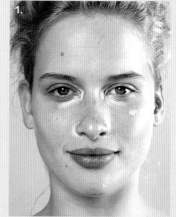
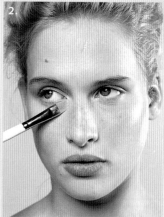
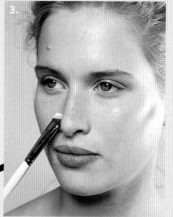
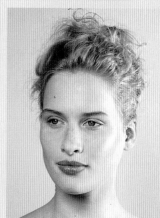

A more sophisticated finish

Step 1 Apply a cream base by rubbing a damp sponge over the base then blending outwards from the center of the face.

Step 2 Apply concealer over the base to the inner corner of the eyes, under the eyes and on any imperfections, making sure to blend well so there are no demarcation lines, especially if your concealer is lighter than your base.

Step 3 Using a powder puff, lightly apply a mat powder all over the face with a soft-but-firm pressing movement, then dust off excess with a large brush. This will make for a longer-lasting makeup.

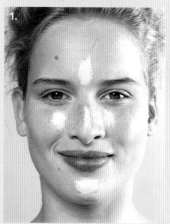
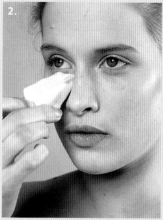
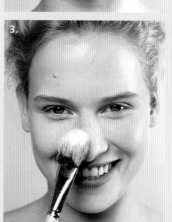
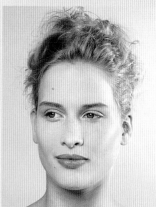

Bruno Gaget (all photos this page).

brows Defining and Shaping

Of all the facial features, the eyebrows are among the most expressive and subtle. They reveal details not only of one's fashion sensibility, but also of one's personality, humor, and wit. The brilliant Mexican painter Frida Kahlo's untamed eyebrows hint at her vibrant, revolutionary spirit, just as chanteuse and film legend Marlene Dietrich's provocative, high-arching brows personify her unnerving self-assurance and brashness. Brooke Shields' full, thick brows made her distinct and exotic at a time when thin-plucked brows were in vogue.

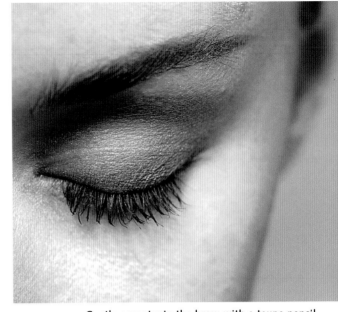

Gently accentuate the brow with a taupe pencil.
Photo by Bruno Gaget.

Note the softer and sharper edges of these two pairs of tweezers. Softer edges are gentler.

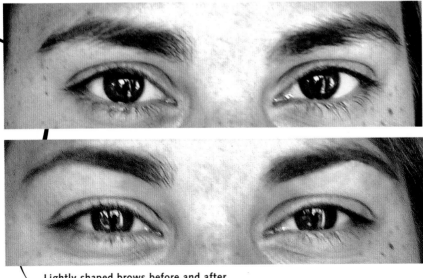

Lightly shaped brows before and after.

Plucking

When most of us started plucking our brows as teenagers, we wanted to emulate whatever look was "in" at the time; we imitated what looked good on others. As your sense of self develops and you gain more confidence in who *you* are and what *you* like, you can start to use your brows as an affirmation of your personality and sense of style. Lifting and shaping the brows through plucking or waxing is one of the simplest ways to streamline your look and neaten up your face. It is a major "pick-me-up" for any woman, no matter what her age. A slight arch can give a face freshness and youthfulness, but be careful: going overboard with the arch can transform you into Cruella Deville.

Plucking can be painful, so choose tweezers with slightly rounded, softer edges—these are gentler. Tweezers don't need to be sharp to exert a good grip. To test their precision, try using them on the hairs of your hand. Run your finger along the tweezer's edges to make sure they're soft.

If you decide you want to pluck your eyebrows, your aim should be to create a soft arch above the center of your eye and to gently taper the brow at the end by plucking and neatening it underneath. Plucking on top could destroy the brow's natural arch. Maintain the space between your eyebrows according to the width and symmetry of your face. If you are wary about plucking your own brows, go to a professional. He or she can show you a style that you can then maintain yourself. If you have heavy brows, do them a little every day over a period of a week to lessen the risk of irritation and of plucking more than you intended. Each of your eyebrows is usually slightly different than the other; look at each carefully, and work a little on each alternately. Always pluck in the direction of the hair, and stretch the skin tight with the forefinger and middle finger of the hand opposite to the one holding the tweezers to avoid plucking the skin or pulling it with the hair. Simply removing the less perceptible hairs under the brow on the eyebrow bone makes an enormous difference and gives your eyes a lift.

Classic plucking method

Before plucking your brows, make sure they don't have any makeup on them. Then there are five points to check.

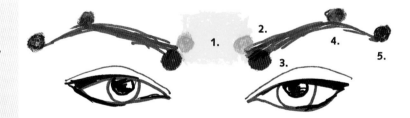

1. **Between the brows** Clean all hairs away from the yellow area.
2. **The beginning of the brows** Ask yourself, are the brows close together? Your eyebrow should begin near the inside corner of your eye. Don't pluck here yet! The brows may look better slightly closer together. You should go back to this point after you have finished the rest.
3. **Under the brows, at the beginning of the brow** Are the brows squishing down here? Do you look like you have a slight frown? If so, open up the eyes by plucking the small hairs from under here; this is especially good for an older woman.
4. **The apex (highest point)** Hold a pencil vertically from the center of your cheekbone through the outer corners of your eye. Then hold it horizontally along your eyebrow. Put a red pencil dot just above your brow at this point. This is the highest point of a perfectly formed, classically arched brow. An arch further out will give a more sophisticated look.
5. **The outer point of the brows** This is where the classic brow should end. Begin plucking here under the brow, tapering them to a point.

Shaping and Coloring

If you have blonde or gray hair and your brows are also light, choose a fairly hard, light-colored eyebrow pencil with a neutral undertone (no red).

You can use this same type of pencil no matter what your coloring to create a neutral "frame" or shape for the brow, which can then be "filled in," or darkened by using pencil or powder in another color. (I'll explain exactly how in "Defining Your Brows.") If you have dark hair, or if you would just like a more dramatic brow, you can add brown or black. Redheads look great with a touch of red-brown color in their brows, and people who have gray hair and dark brows can dust in a little gray for softness.

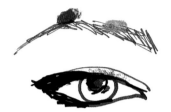 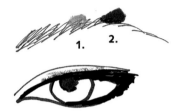

To make the eyebrows more arched, make sure they are well-penciled in at point 1 and point 2. Keep the penciling in the upper part of the brows at this point.

Defining Your Brows

With the right product and technique, you can completely change your look by defining the arch of your brow. To fill in empty spaces or define the arch (or other parts of the brow that might need strengthening), I recommend that you begin with a pencil. The tip gives you more control over where the color goes as well as the ability to add definition in small areas; you can then finish off with an eyebrow or eye shadow powder.

You can define your brows by just drawing a line with an eyebrow pencil, either along the edge of or in the area you want to define, but this will not give a natural effect. Make short, sharp lines in the same direction the hair naturally grows, then brush the lines with your eyebrow brush to soften them. Another method is to gently rub the pencil on the skin, pushing the hairs against the way they grow, then brush the brows with your eyebrow brush to shape them and soften the color. If you then press translucent powder onto the brow using a firm eyeshadow brush or a powder puff, the eyepencil-color will last longer. Brush the brows again with your eyebrow brush to remove any excess powder, then apply a little brow gel to tame them.

If you want to give your brows a slight color change but don't want to alter their shape or fill in any empty spaces, you can do any of the following: Brush on an eyebrow or eye shadow powder with a firm-haired, angled eye shadow brush. Then, lightly rub an eyebrow pencil back and forth on the hair of the brows. Brush on a clear gel with either an eyebrow brush or mascara wand.

Tools

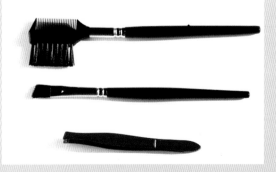

1. A brush to tame the brows and remove excess color, base, and powder.
2. An angled brush for applying powder or cake-color to the brows.
3. Tweezers.

eyes

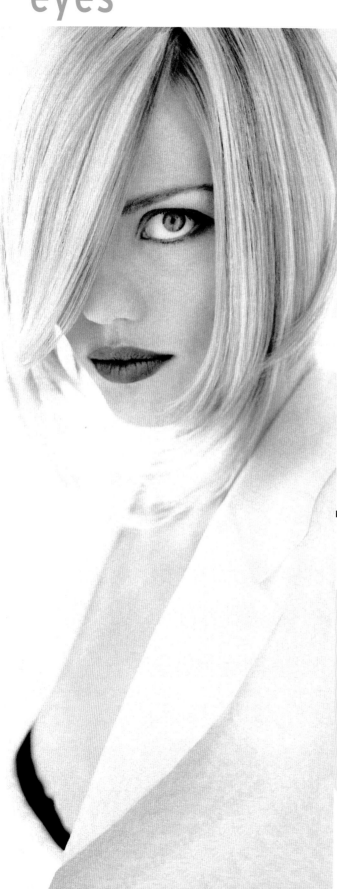

When I was in a model agency one day, I noticed all the models' headshots hanging on the wall. I looked at all the photos together, and I immediately understood the saying, "Eyes are windows of the soul." Each girl's eyes seemed to jump out at me, and what she was *truly* feeling at the moment her picture was taken became clear to me, no matter what emotion she may have been trying to project for the camera. Even if the model had managed to produce a twinkle of joy for the photo, if she were feeling any sadness on a deeper level, I could sense it in her eyes. This communicative quality is what makes eyes beautiful. Makeup can enhance, enlarge, or emphasize eyes and make them even more intense and expressive.

A soft, smoky eye with a defined lip—very '90s.
Photo by Diego Uchitel.
Hair: John Sahag.

Eye Shadow

Eye shadow comes in a variety of textures: there are matte powder, semi-matte, pearl (iridescent), cream, and gel eye shadows. If you have perfectly smooth lids, you can wear all of these textures. If your lid is not so smooth, you should stick with the matte and semi-matte powders because pearls, creams, and gels will accentuate lines and creases. However, if you want to try pearl powder or cream shadow, you can use a very slight hint on the smoother parts of your lid (just under the brow or in the inner corner of the eye, right next to the lash line).

Using creams and powders together is also a good idea. You can intensify the powders by applying creams to the lid first. You should apply translucent powder after you apply a creamy cosmetic (eye shadow, blush, base) if you want its effects to last a long time. If you leave an eye cream or gloss sticky or shiny, you can add a nice effect like glitter onto the lid and it will stay put. Be careful not to put it next to the eye. Gels tend to give a more transparent coverage on the lid and will keep a slight shine if that is the effect you are looking for; they will not stay wet and they are longer-lasting, but they are more difficult to blend with other colors or textures.

Textures

1. Pencils are good for lining and deepening the eyes. Make sure they are soft and easy to blend.

2. Creams can be used alone for a light color wash or under powders to deepen or brighten them.

3. Light powders will bring out the eyes.

4. Matte or dark powders will deepen or shape the eyes and set pencil liner.

5. Cake (add water to these), liquid, and gel liners allow you to strengthen the eyes further and make a makeup more sophisticated.

6. Gloss.

7. Glitter.

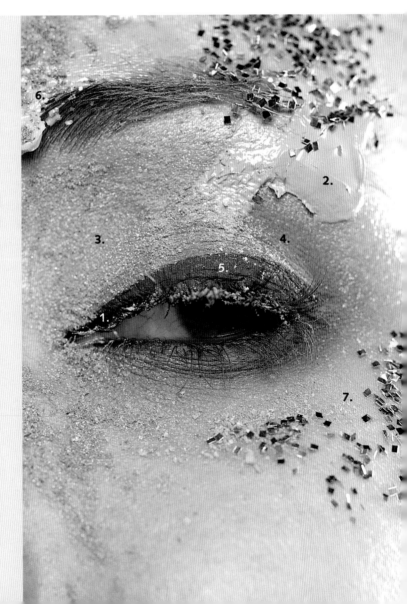

Photo by Bruno Gaget.

Applying Eye Shadow

It is not always necessary to even out the skin tone of your eyelid before applying eye shadow. If your eyelids have a slight natural coloring, they can be a great canvas for a soft, natural eye makeup. If your lid has a slight yellow/green undertone, just add a highlight to the center of the lid using an iridescent ivory shadow. If your lid has a pink undertone, use an iridescent lilac shadow. Then apply a deeper soft matte shade in the same color family (ivory or lilac), such as a yellow-toned brown with the ivory or a pinky-brown with the lilac shade, like a liner next to the lashes near the lash line, to give a little depth. If your eyes are deep-set or the skin of your eyelids is dark, applying a special neutral eye shadow base (or a little regular base or concealer) will give you a lighter "canvas" to work on, and it will be easier for you to blend your eye shadow colors.

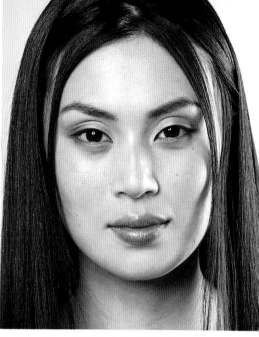

Two-toned eye, lightly shaded. Blend a soft, demi-pearl shadow over your eyelid to create a soft, smooth, lightly shaded lid; then add a touch of a lighter, more iridescent shadow under the brow bone and next to the pupil at the base of the lashes to highlight and give a little more depth.
Photo by Bruno Gaget. Hair: Mayumi for John Sahag.

Knowing which colors will give light and which will give depth is important. If you have two colors you want to apply to your eyes, the darker color (even if it's only a fraction darker and especially if it's matte) will give an impression of depth when it's next to the lighter color. However, this is not true if the color is very iridescent. If you have two colors that appear to be the same depth of color but one of them is iridescent, that color will attract the light (especially in photos) and therefore appear lighter. When choosing eye-shadow colors, apply them next to each other on your inner forearm and move your arm around in the light to see how the eye shadow reflects it and how the color lightens. If, however, you apply an iridescent color in a concave area such as the inner corner of your eyelid or under the eye, beware: it will make the area look more concave. If you have close- or deep-set eyes, it's not a good idea to apply iridescent shadow in these deeper, more recessed areas (see pages 48–49).

If you have evenly spaced eyes and smooth lids, you can do just about anything with eye shadow and pull it off, but the majority of women have something that they would like to play down or bring out. Many aren't sure how to go about it, but in the majority of cases, it is just a matter of the positioning of the shadow and eyeliner; the sketches on pages 48–49 explain how.

There are two methods of applying powder eye shadows: **"a cote,"** which means applying one shade of shadow next to the other so that the lighter color is accentuated and the darker deepened, and **"layered,"** which means adding touches of other colors to a base color.

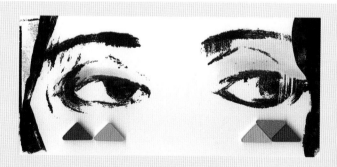

A Cote: Keeping bright colors next to the eye instead of right up to the eyebrow makes them much easier to wear.

Layered: Layering a bright color onto a softer, earthier tone is a good way to start for someone afraid of color. First apply a shade like gold or a soft brown or beige to the lid, then add touches of color to highlight.

Eye Shadow Looks

1. For close-set eyes, do not go right into the inner corner of the eyes with darker shadows or liner.

2. For eyes with a heavy fold or just to lift the eyes further, apply a lot of deeper shadow in the crease of the eye at the outer corner and blend it over the eye bone past the crease.

3. To lengthen the eyes, make your shading much stronger in the outer corner of the eye and keep it very thin under and over the pupil (the center of the eye).

4. To make the eyes more intense, apply black pencil over the color already applied into the very base of the lashes.

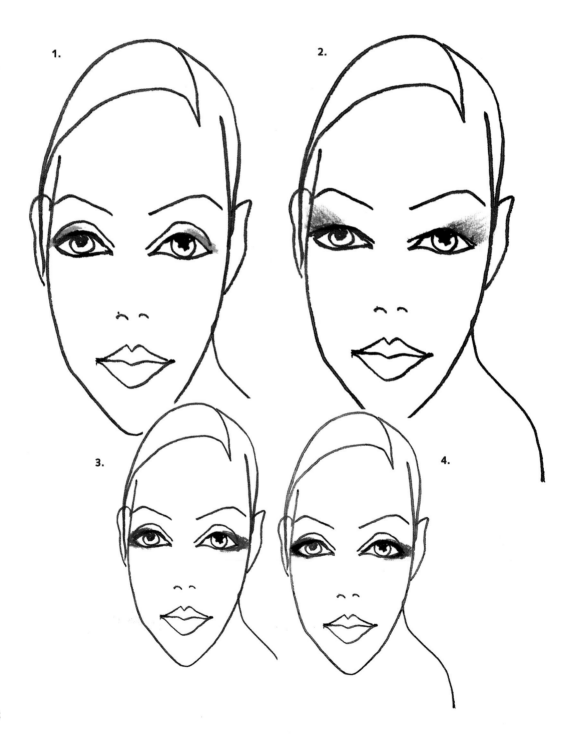

5. Add touches of light to the center of the eyelid next to the pupil to brighten the eye. These touches of light can be made with a paler shade or a brighter shade.

6. To make the eye rounder, draw the shading thicker in the center of the eye, above and below the eye.

7. Add shine or a light shade of powder under the eyebrows to deepen the eye.

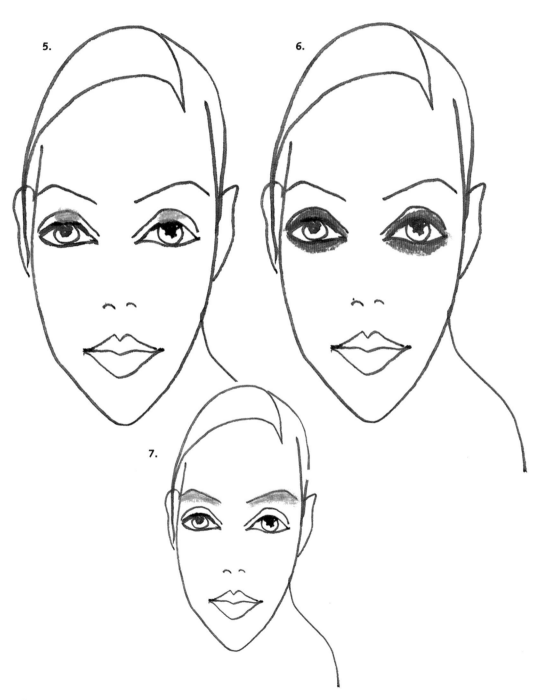

What Color Eye Shadow to Wear

Throughout the years I have been asked by magazine editors to help give women a set formula for choosing eye shadow colors that "go with" their coloring. I find this very difficult; each person is different, and individual personality and fashion play an important role in what color "works" for you. A reserved but smoldering personality would probably be best expressed with a dark, smoky eye, whereas an outgoing, vivacious type might look best in a light, bright eye shadow or soft, natural eye makeup and a brighter lip color. However, most women are many things—the joy of makeup is in its power to transform. I encourage you to experiment with any eye color to which you are drawn. When you are drawn to a particular color, it's probably because it expresses some aspect of your mood or personality. If you want to wear blue, try as many blues as you like and you will eventually find the right shade. When you are experimenting, wear clothes in a neutral color and no lipstick so you don't have any colors to interfere with or distract you from making the right choice.

Life is in perpetual motion. We evolve, our hair color changes, our skin tone changes, and the kind of light around us can make our hair and skin look different. Therefore, it is only natural that we should seek change in our makeup. When I go on photo shoots, we sometimes have to change one model's eye-makeup colors three or four times; as a makeup artist, it is my job to make sure she looks good in all of those colors. There are things you can do to make whatever kind of eye makeup you wear look better. Evening out the imperfections in your skin tone so they don't distract attention from your eyes strengthens their impact and makes it easier for you to wear a larger variety of eye-shadow colors. Keeping bright colors right next to the eye instead of near the eyebrows works best. That way, the color accents your eye color. If you are a bit afraid of color, but also a bit curious, try layering a brighter color onto an earthier one. The bright color then acts as a subtle highlight. You can layer one color over another to alter the shape of the eye slightly, or two colors over another to shape it more.

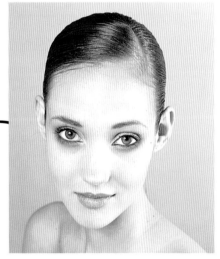

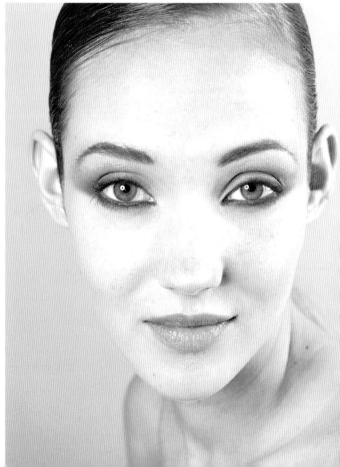

Although Abby does not have deep-set eyes, she has a rather long narrow face. By keeping the inner corner of the eye light and lengthening the shadow in the outer corner, as shown here, you can create the impression of more width in the face and wider spaced eyes. The shadows are blended around the eye to make the eyes appear rounder. In the photo on the right, I lengthened the eyes by blending the deeper shadow outward. *Photos by Bruno Gaget.*

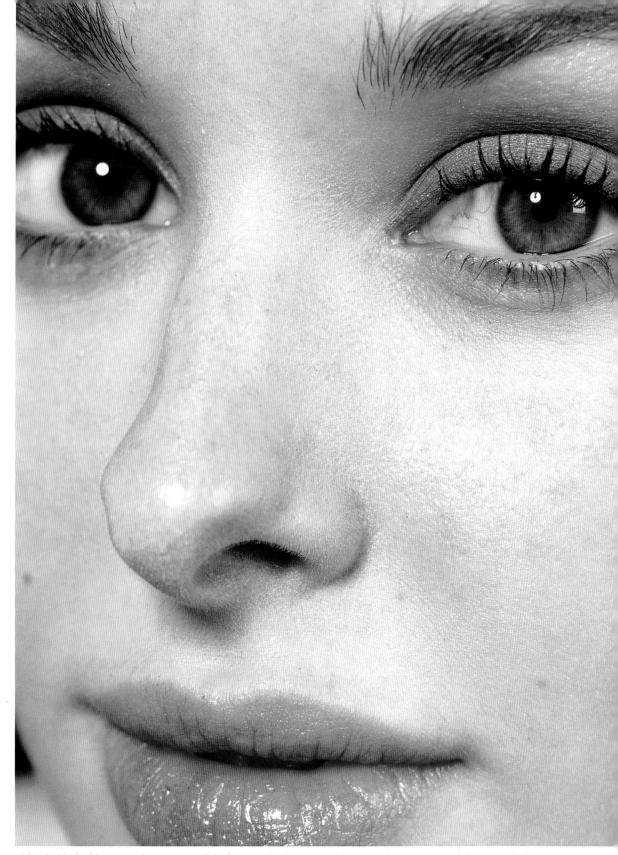

I blended light blue over the entire eyelid, then used a blue pencil liner on the very base of the upper lashes to give depth and blended the line slightly with a small brush. A deeper shade of blue eye shadow was then blended over the pencil liner from the base of the upper lashes outwards and upwards. *Photo by Bruno Gaget for* Good Housekeeping, *2001.*

Eye Shadow Brushes

Good eye shadow and liner brushes should last a long time—even with frequent washing. If you have a tendency to go backwards and forwards with the brush, you will need a soft, fluffy one. This is also the case if you use the side of the brush; a firmer brush's bristles could irritate your lid. I apply shadows by blending them with the flat side of the brush, (always "sweeping" in the same direction). Because I use powder eye shadows that are more compact, I like firm, tapered brushes. When applying my own eye shadow, I sometimes use sponge-tipped applicators. Keep your brushes clean by washing and rinsing them thoroughly with hot water. Don't use the same brush for your light and dark colors. Keep a larger brush for lighter colors that you apply over larger areas of the lid, and use the smaller-headed brushes for darker shadows you use in smaller areas. If you use more than one color on the same brush, flick the hair of your brush to eliminate the first color before applying the second, and don't apply powdered eye shadow with a brush over eye makeup that has grease in it, such as a pencil or cream. This will get on the brush and make the powder blotchy and heavy and will also create a film, making it more difficult to use. Use synthetic brushes for creams or gels and natural hair for powder shadows.

Tools

1. Use this large-headed, firm brush to quickly dust over the lids with transparent powder or a soft, light shade of shadow.

2. Another good eye-shadow brush for larger areas of the lid.

3. This brush is good for blending shadows together, especially over the mobile part of the eyelid.

4. This smaller, slightly fluffier brush is good for blending deeper colors of shadow into the crease of the lid or in smaller areas of the lid.

5. A small firm brush is great for blending pencil liner at the base of the lashes or shadows in the crease of the eye.

6. This very small liner brush is good for getting into the base of the lashes with pencils, powders, and cake eyeliner.

7. The synthetic hair of this brush makes it suitable for blending cream shadows.

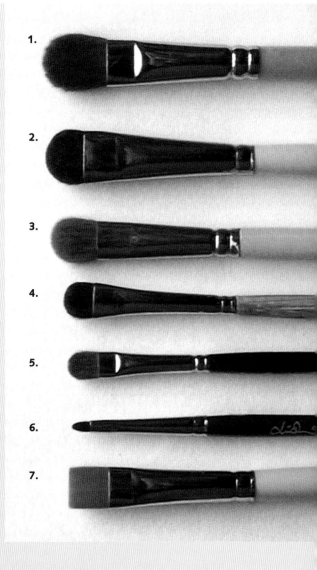

1.

2.

3.

4.

5.

6.

7.

Eyeliner

If you use an eye pencil to line your eyes, it should be soft and well sharpened. Try the pencil on your hand. If you have to press hard to get color, it is not a good choice for lining. The good thing about using an eye pencil is that you can blend the line to soften it. It is also easy to apply to the base of the lower lashes, and you can apply powdered shadow over it.

Gel, cake, and liquid liners will give you more strength and intensity. If you work quickly, you can blend the edge of the line slightly for a softer effect. With a cake liner, you can easily see the amount you have on your brush; then, if you want a heavier line, you can just mix it to a heavier paste. Eyeliner does not need to be seen to be effective. By just lifting the eyelid gently and rubbing a little bit of creamy pencil into the very base of the upper, outer lashes, you can give the eye strength and lift. This is a quick, effective way to lightly define the eyes without shadows or other products.

Unless you are very adept, it is safest to begin applying any type of eyeliner in the outer, upper corner of the eyelid; this is where the liner should be the heaviest, unless you want to give your eyes a downturn. If so, apply a very thin line from the inner corner of the eye to join with the line from the outer corner, making sure that the liner is very thin over the pupil. Make sure you look straight ahead with your face relaxed when you are applying liner so you can see the shape you are giving the eye. If you want to make the shape of your eye more round, line the inner corner and over the pupil more thickly. It is still important to keep the liner in the outer corner a fraction thicker.

To give a natural lift to your eyes, before or after you apply any colored shadows, blend a little gray or brown pencil into the very base of the upper lashes in the outer, upper corner of the eyes. Make sure to apply the pencil into the very base of the lashes as shown.

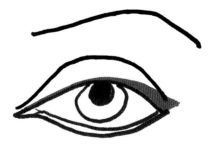

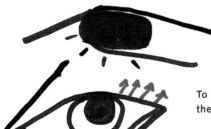

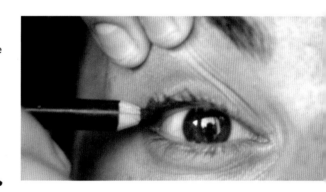

To apply eyeliner, first gently pull the skin of the lid upwards.

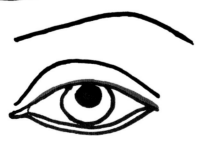

Apply a very thin line right in the base of the lashes, beginning at the outer corner and working inwards.

You can then thicken the liner in the outer corner of the eye.

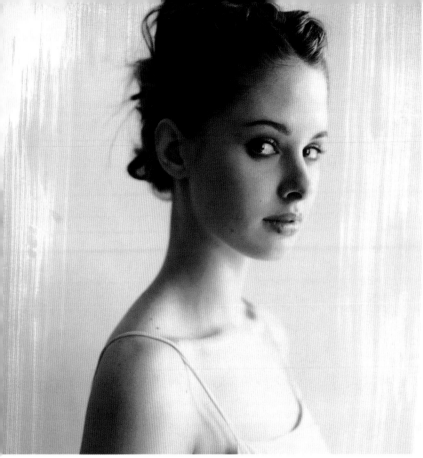

Here, the upper and lower lashes are lightly defined with blended pencil liner.

Photo by Patrick Demarchelier. Hair: John Sahag. Model: Trish.

Mascara Black mascara is not necessarily only for brunettes—it is for anyone who wants to make her eyes more intense. Brown creates a softer effect. Green and blue mascara can brighten the face; subtly colored mascaras such as these are a great pick-me-up for someone with delicate features who doesn't like to wear colored shadow or strong lip color.

If you are a blonde or a redhead and would like a very soft effect, try not wearing mascara at all. If you're a brunette and you want a soft effect, a touch of brown or gray pencil in the base of the lashes is a gentler way of strengthening them than wearing mascara.

Many people do not apply their mascara into the very base of their lashes. If your lashes are dark, it doesn't matter so much, but if your lashes are light, the lack of mascara at the base creates a light space between the lashes and the eyeliner and distorts the shape of the eye makeup. By wiggling the mascara wand from side to side at the base of the lashes, then applying the rest by placing the wand in the base of the lashes and gently moving it from side to side while working it through to the tips with a back and forth motion, you should be able to color the base of the lashes.

cheeks Choice and Texture of Blush

Rouge placement can totally change the rest of your face and—if you're not careful—very much date a look. Many times I recommend that women change the kind of blush she uses. The wrong product can just sit on the skin and make it appear dull, whereas choosing a different color or choosing a cream rather than a powder can brighten up the whole face.

Using the right type of blush can both soften the shape of a face and lighten and brighten it. It can give you a warm radiance or a sultry, sculptured look. If you have clear skin and would like to give your face a natural, healthy glow, choose a gel or cream. I prefer creams because I like to mix colors or add powders to complete a look, and that is easier to do with creams. If you don't have clear skin, it is usually better to use a powder blush. I add a touch of powder blush over cream blush to create a more finished look (you will find that powder blushes are easier to apply on powdered skin). If you apply just a little at a time, you can brighten up your cream by brushing the powder blush gently onto unpowdered skin. Pearl blushers give extra highlight when added to convex areas of the face such as the cheekbones, but when they are applied to hollow areas, they will accentuate discoloration and depth.

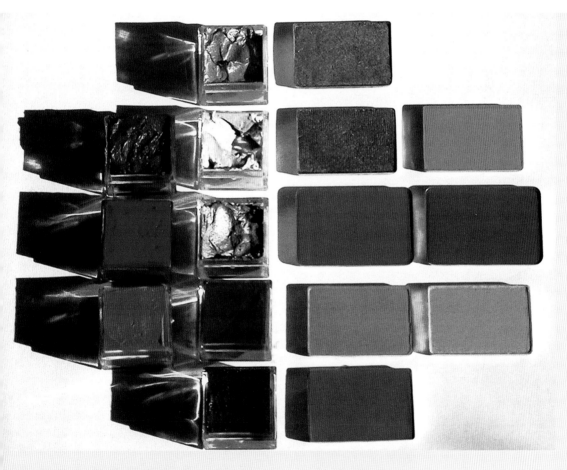

Blush Products

1. Transparent creams and gels are good for a natural glow. You need fairly clear skin to wear these.
2. Powders can be used alone, but are more easily to apply over a powdered skin. Used carefully, they can be added to creams to strengthen them.
3. All pearls applied to convex areas of the face will give extra highlight and emphasis to these areas, but on concave areas, such as the under-eye area, will accentuate discoloration and depth.

Don't be afraid of bright, pure, clean colors of blush; whether it's powder, cream, or gel, a pure, strong color tends to blend in with the natural skin tone and just brighten the face slightly. What may look too strong or vibrant in the packaging can look natural and soft on your face. You must apply such colors delicately and sparingly, however; you don't want to end up looking like a doll with bright red cheeks. But a fresh, pure, strong pink blush applied delicately will blend with the oils of your skin and give you a wonderful, rosy glow. The pure, strong colors can actually end up being more natural-looking than those that look more neutral, muted and "natural" in the package—such shades tend to have a lot of gray in the pigment, which tends to dull the skin.

As you should do with your base, try them on the inner side of your forearm to see what they do to your skin. Something that looks natural in the tube or in the compact may make your skin look dull when it's actually applied. One of my two favorite colors is a clean, light-pink cream blush; it is very natural on fair skin but can also look natural on some olive complexions—it gives them a slight lift. My other favorite is a red-brown cream blush because it blends well on all skin tones, giving darker skin a natural glow and fair skin a ruddy, fresh appearance. I often use these two together; for an evening look, I add a powder blush to heighten the color. If you are applying a powder blush over a cream blush, keep in mind that the oils of the cream blush will make whichever color powder you choose a little darker than it would look applied by itself. Use a lighter shade of powder blush to avoid this darkening of color, unless that's the look you want.

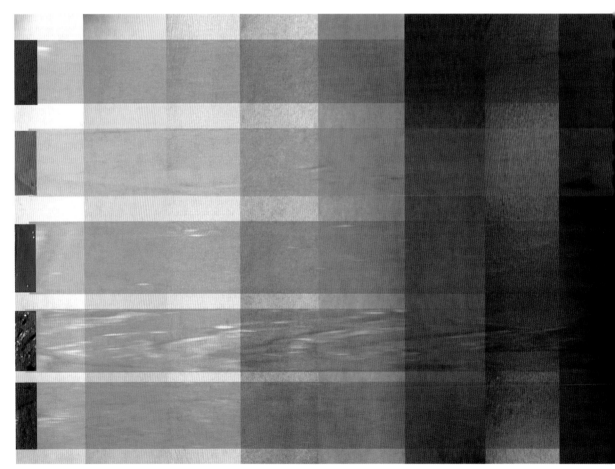

Applying different colors of cream blush (shown on the far left and running in horizontal stripes) on a range of skin tones from light to dark (running in vertical stripes, starting from left). To see how a particular color of cream blush would look on your skin, choose your approximate skin tone from one of the vertical columns, then, going from top to bottom, see how the colors represented on the left will look on that color skin.

Blush Placement

The placement of your blush can affect the overall look of your makeup. You can give strong eyes and lips a softer feel by applying a soft, light blush color on the apples of your cheeks, or you can reinforce the sophisticated look of your strong eye and lip color by applying your blush under your cheekbones in a slanted manner. Many women have difficulty figuring out what their exact face shape is, but that's okay—it's not that important. What is important is to understand how positioning your blush can enhance or soften certain facial features. Applying blush on the apple of the cheek will soften a face with lots of angles, and positioning blush on the underside of the cheekbone and blending downwards on a slant will make a face that's very round look a little more angled. If you have a narrow face and a large nose, placing your blusher on your face widely, farther away from your nose, takes the attention away from your nose. Positioning the blusher horizontally makes a long face look shorter.

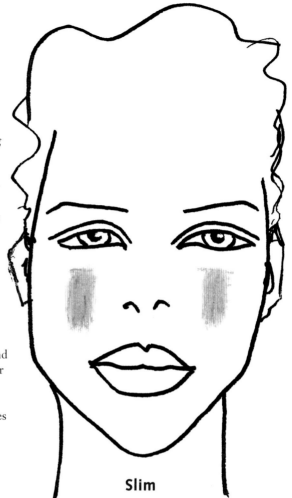

Slim

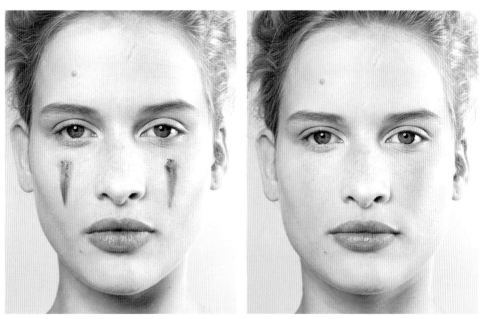

Placing the blush vertically in a narrow line down the center of each cheek will make a rather large face look slimmer. *Photos by Bruno Gaget. Hair: Mayumi for John Sahag.*

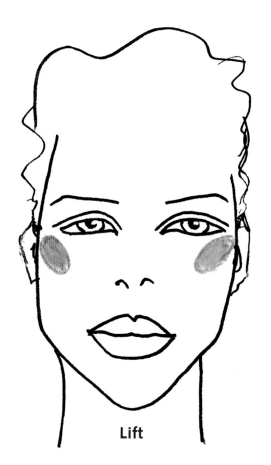

Lift

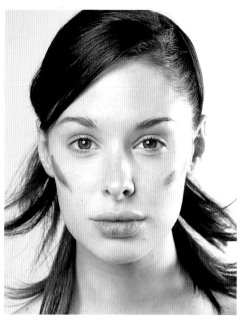

Lift To accentuate good cheek-bones, give the impression of having them, or to just give the face a lift, apply blush high on the cheekbone near the eyes.

Photos (both pages) by Bruno Gaget. Hair: Mayumi for John Sahag.

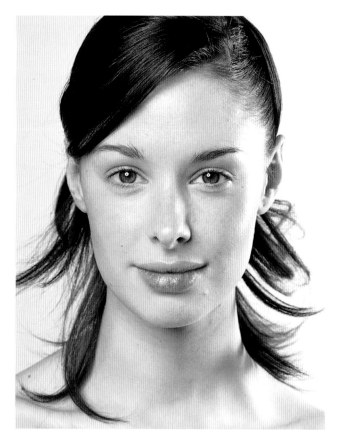

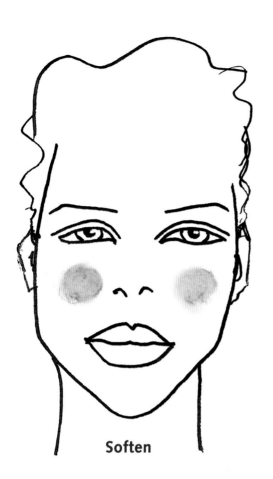

Soften

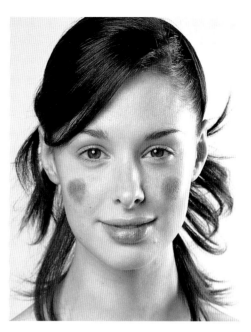

Soften To accentuate a fresh face, place blush on the apples of the cheeks.

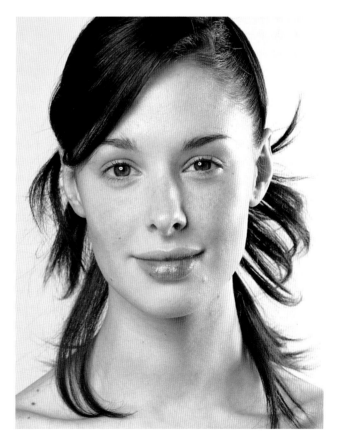

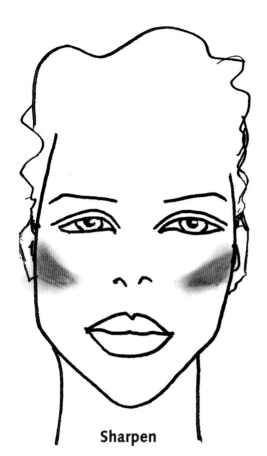

Sharpen

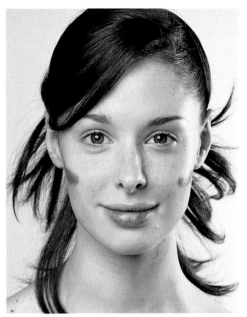

Place the blush under the bone to accentuate the cheekbones.

Sharpen To make your face more angular. Do not do this placement too low, just on the underside of the bone.

When blended, this blush placement will give you a more sophisticated appearance.
Photos by Bruno Gaget.
Hair: John Sahag.

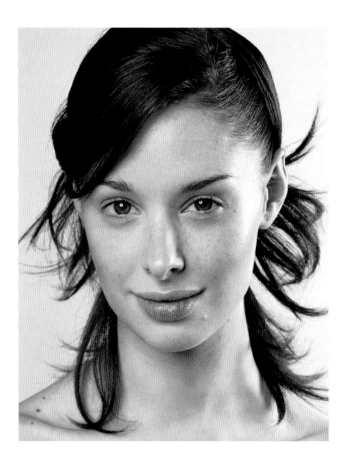

Widen To reduce the length of
a long narrow face, do all blush
placements more horizontally.

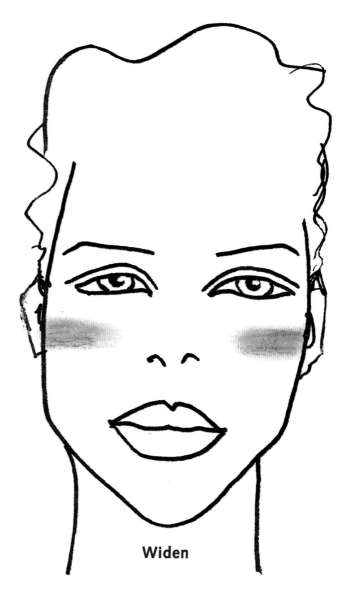

Widen

What to Use to Apply Blush

For the best control over cream blush,
apply it with your fingers. Apply a dot
of color to the area where you would
like the color to be the most intense,
and then blend it well. A small, shaped
blusher brush will give you the best
control when applying a powder blush;
the movement you make with the
brush should be smooth, and you
should always move it in the same
direction. If you go back and forth with
the brush, you could irritate your skin.
A large, soft, floppy brush is better for
applying powder that way.

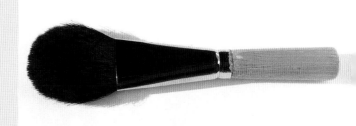

This medium-sized, oval, tapered brush allows for a good positioning of powder blush and/or
contouring powder. To apply cream blush, use a sponge or your fingers. To accentuate a fresh face,
place blush on the apples of the cheeks.

lips

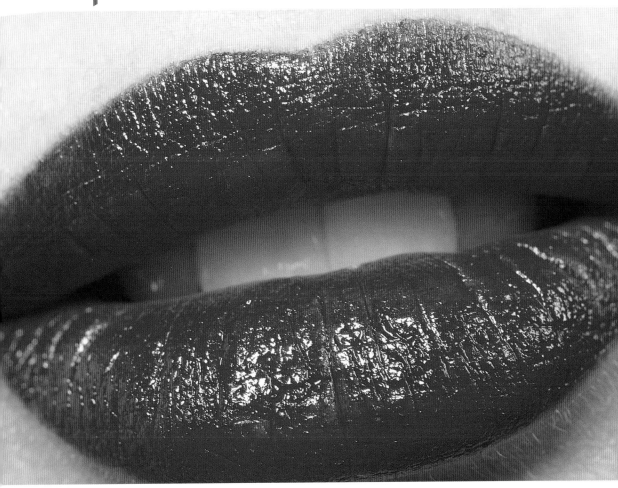

Perfect cherry-red lips. *Photo by Bruno Gaget.*

The lips are the pivotal point of the face. A great lip color can bring light and focus to a woman's features, and, of course, highlight her smile. It doesn't matter whether lips are well-defined with lipstick and lipliner or just smeared with gloss, wearing lip color is the quickest, simplest way to alter the way one's whole face looks.

As a makeup artist, I'm always getting requests from clients to make their lips look fuller. Yes, full lips have been fashionable for quite some time now, and they can be beautiful, but smaller lips can be just as appealing and sexy. The sense of harmony created by having all the other facial features look good in unison is what is important, that is the look you are trying to project. The idea behind the art of beauty is to *use what you've got and have fun with it*. For example, I recently gave a client two makeup lessons a few weeks apart. The first time she came in to see me, she was projecting a smart but conventional image and wearing a gray suit. She had undefined, rather small lips, and I enlarged them with a pencil, building them up in a conventional manner. It worked, and she looked great. When she returned for her next class about a month later, she was wearing softer, fresher colors and conveyed a totally different feel. Giving her lips definition with a pencil the way I had done before did not work with the change in her appearance, and after a little experimenting, we realized she needed a softer, undefined lip to accentuate the softness in her clothes and mood.

Choice and Texture of Lip Color

One of the most exciting things about being a makeup artist is that you get to shop as much as you want for cosmetics without feeling guilty about spending too much time and money on makeup. As a makeup artist during the '70s, I spent a lot of my time searching for the perfect lipstick. To me, that meant a lip color that had the same intensity on the lips as it had in the wand and a color that stayed on. Lipsticks in the '70s were very glossy, so it was impossible to find one that didn't run. I found some great lipsticks from the '40s in a little shop in Milan—called Perfumeria Ditta Bianchi—and *voila*! These lipsticks wouldn't budge, and they were as intense on the lips as they were in the wand. To create matte shades, which were totally impossible to find, I would press crumbled eye-shadow powder in bright colors onto the glossier lipsticks. To this day, I still prefer to work with more heavily pigmented lipsticks. When I created my makeup line, I made sure that the lip colors were pure and heavily pigmented; these are best for anyone who wants to mix his or her own color or give volume and definition to their lips. You can still create a light effect by just rubbing a little color lightly on the lips with your fingertip. For shine, apply gloss.

Textures of lip color (clockwise from top left): matte, creamy; stain; pearl. *Photo by Bruno Gaget.*

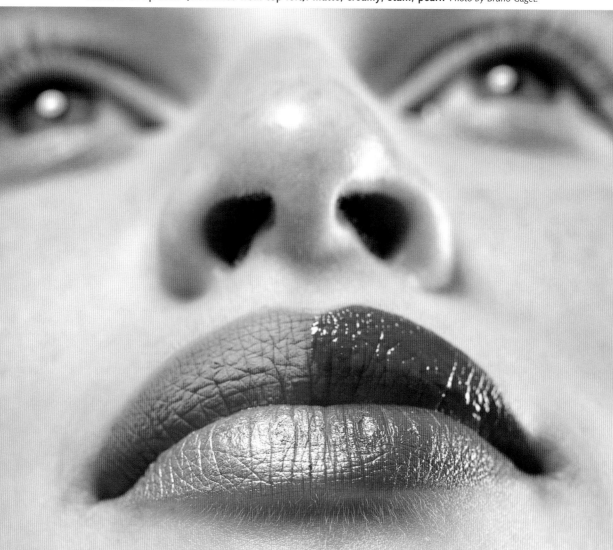

How to Apply Lip Color

Always prime your lips before applying lip color. This does not mean applying lip salve; the models with whom I work who apply this many times during the course of the day have lips in the worst condition. Just rub them gently with a wet cotton swab to remove any dead skin or makeup base. For dry lips, I often apply a little lip gloss and then wipe it off before applying lipstick. If you have a fever blister, dry it as much as you can with a Kleenex, apply Dermablend (a great scar concealer) gently with a brush, then gently apply lip color, also using a brush.

To strengthen your lips, start by applying the lip color either with a tube or brush, then use your lip brush to work the lip color right to the edge of the lips from the center outwards. Then define them even more by using a lip pencil the same shade as the lip color around the outline, blending into the lip color. For a softer lip line, instead of using a pencil, use a slightly deeper lip color. Layering color makes lips look fuller and gives the impression of depth and volume. It is different from mixing, which just gives you a larger variety of colors.

To set your lip color, blot the lips, then powder around the edge with a large-headed, clean shadow brush. Another tip for setting the lipstick is to put a little loose powder inside a Kleenex and gently press the Kleenex on your lips. For further staying power, seal your lips with a lip-fixing product.

Many women with narrow lips feel more comfortable defining their lips with a lip pencil than they do filling in the lips with the pencil color; for defining the lips, the pencil you use should be soft. To take away the harsh effect the liner can give to the edge of the lips, smile and rub the edges lightly with a Kleenex.

To prevent excess lip color from getting on your teeth after applying lipstick, pucker your mouth around your index finger and then pull it back out.

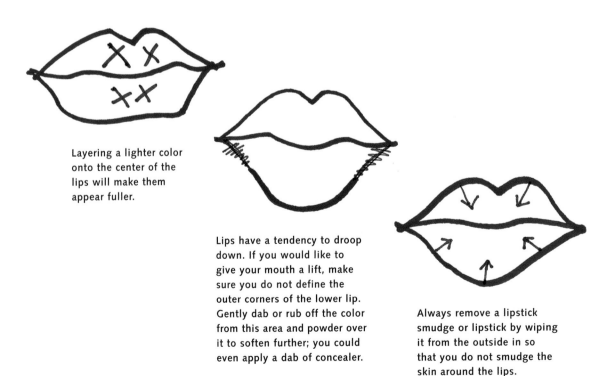

Layering a lighter color onto the center of the lips will make them appear fuller.

Lips have a tendency to droop down. If you would like to give your mouth a lift, make sure you do not define the outer corners of the lower lip. Gently dab or rub off the color from this area and powder over it to soften further; you could even apply a dab of concealer.

Always remove a lipstick smudge or lipstick by wiping it from the outside in so that you do not smudge the skin around the lips.

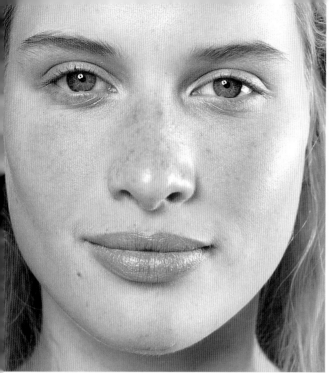

Light

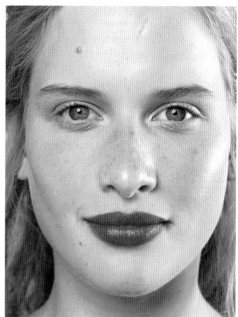

Bright

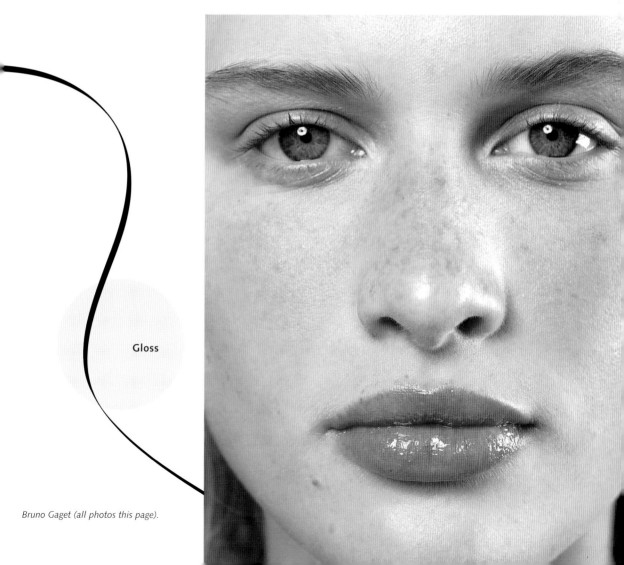

Gloss

Bruno Gaget (all photos this page).

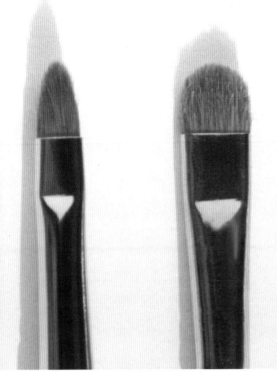

A natural hair brush with a tapered point is the best brush for most women with small to medium-large lips. This brush is also good for defining the edges of very full lips. For very full lips, a wider, flatter brush is easiest to use, especially for filling in the center.

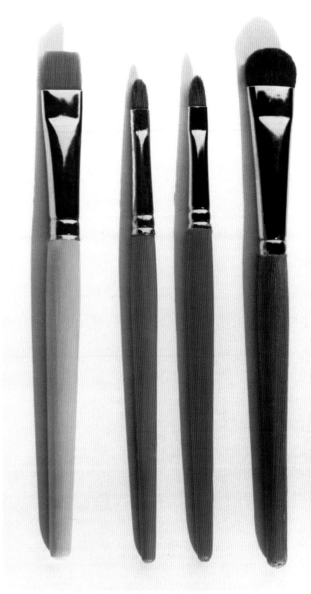

A concealer brush is good for covering any redness you may have around your lips that might distract from their freshness. Lipbrushes with tapered points are essentials for applying color evenly. The same large-headed eye-shadow brush that you used to apply powder over your concealer can be used to soften and set the color around the edges of the lips.

Tools

A good lip brush is essential to achieving a great lip shape. Having the right brush is a great investment and will make lip lining and defining easy. Choose a sable brush that is full and rather flat with a taper, but not too pointed. Women with very full lips should use an eye-shadow brush for filling in color and a smaller lipbrush for contouring.

Mixing Color

The lip colors shown on the right are just some of the shades you can obtain through mixing or layering the three lip colors and the gloss in each of the color palettes in my makeup line.

I include four **basic** colors (numbered 1–4 in the top row of the photo) in each of my color wheels:

1. A brown shade
2. A gloss
3. A pale shade
4. A bright color

You can get four **new** colors (numbered 5–8 in the bottom row of the photo) by mixing and layering the four basic colors from the top row in the following manner:

5. For a bright color, begin with a bright color and only mix other bright colors into the first one. (Mix color 4 with color 2.)

6. If you want a pale color, begin with a pale shade, then add touches of a brighter or a browner shade. (Mix 2 with 3.)

7. Adding a light color to a red will make it pinker. (Mix 4 with 3.)

8. For a dark color, start with the darkest color, e.g., dark brown, then blend in another color such as a ruby. (Mix 4 with 1.)

Wipe your brush between colors.

Many women ask when they should add gloss. Applying your gloss *first*, then adding touches of color will give your lips a softer effect than adding gloss after all your color, unless you have just used a color stain.

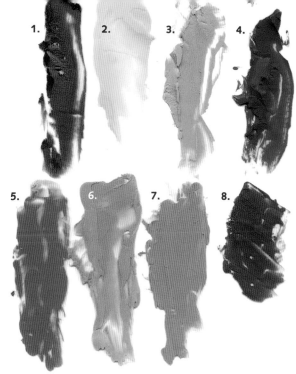

Fire lip colors. Mixing the colors in the top row creates the colors in the bottom row.

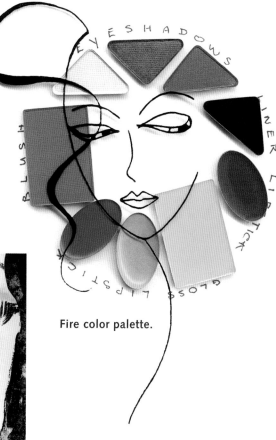

Fire color palette.

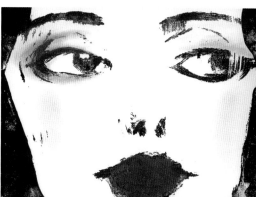

Fire lip and eye colors on a finished face.

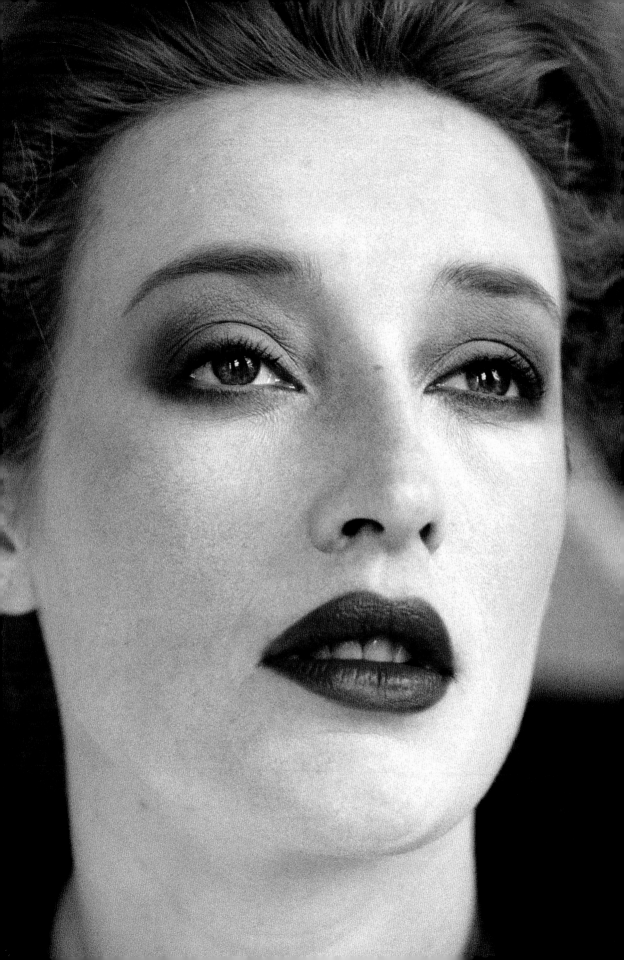

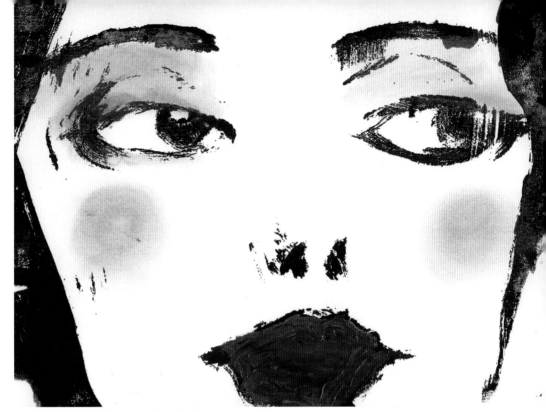

Earth lip and eye colors on a finished face.

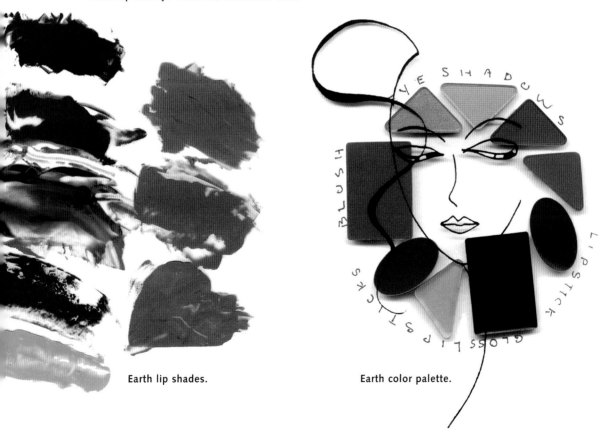

Earth lip shades.

Earth color palette.

OPPOSITE PAGE Model wearing makeup from my Earth color palette, one of four color wheels in my "Harmonies" makeup line, which makes mixing colors easier and faster. Any of the colors in the wheel works together with any other color in the set. In this photo, a layered brown eye shadow is intensified with pencil liner; the lip color is also layered.

putting it all together

As I mentioned before, the enjoyment of makeup is in playing with it, but working within certain guidelines can eliminate some of the guesswork and trial and error.

When beginning your makeup, if having a healthy glow helps give you a sense what will look good on the rest of your face—a sense of balance and placement for the rest of your makeup—then begin with your blush. Trying a new eye color? Begin with it. If you adore lipstick, use your lip color as your starting point. Start with something that inspires you or makes you feel good.

To create a sophisticated finish, I used cream base, blush, powder, and two eye shadows. I blended a white shadow over the entire eyelid and lined the eyes with a dark green liner. I finished the look with a muted pink lipstick. *Photos (both pages) by Michael Myers for YM magazine, 2001.*

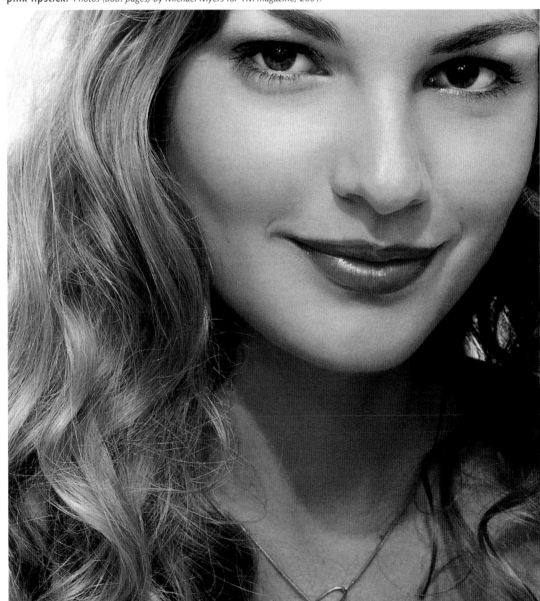

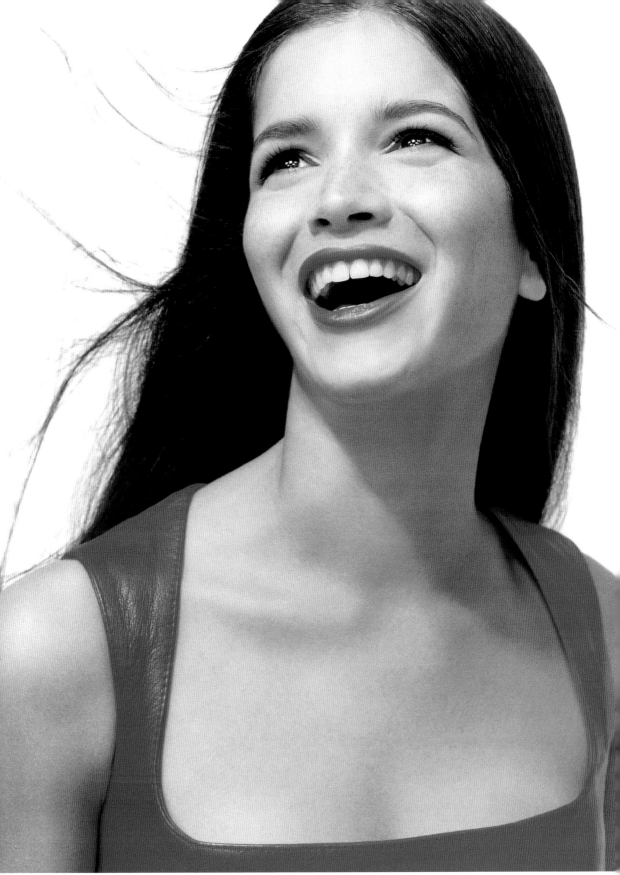

To give this model a look reminiscent of the '50s, I used lots of mascara, eyeliner, and red lip color.

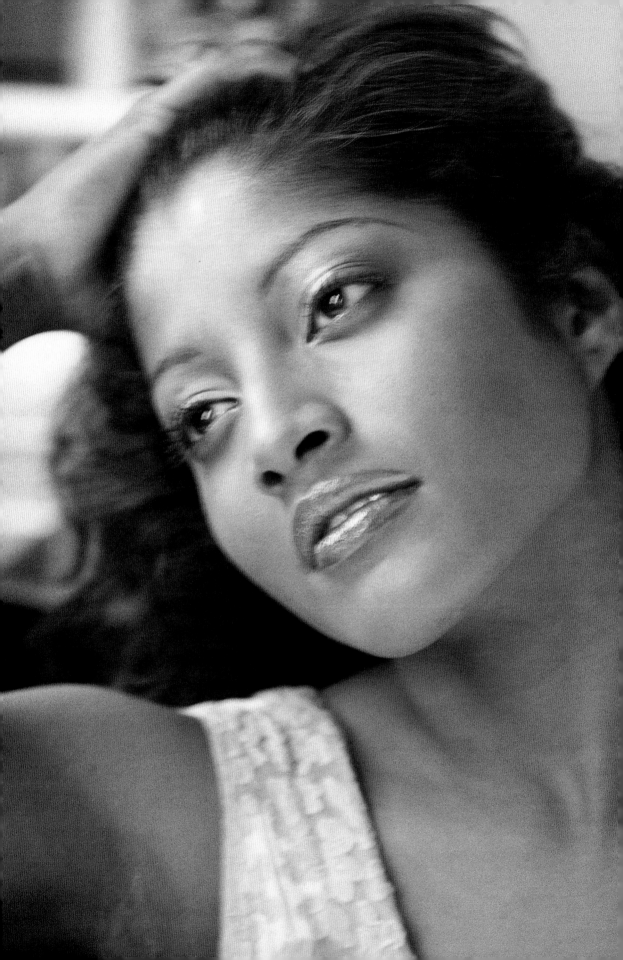

glamourizing techniques

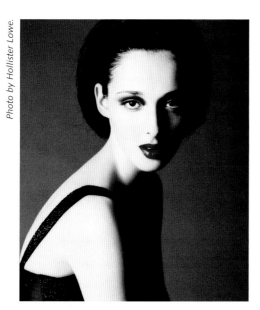

Photo by Hollister Lowe.

Throughout the twentieth century, a decade was rarely defined by only one look. There was, rather, an evolution of looks, styles, and flashes of experimentation that predicted what would become major trends ten years down the line. Thus, elements of what we may consider the classic "look" of the '40s probably had their origins in the styles of a different time, but their combination with other elements in a new context gave them a unique, stand-out effect that took hold.

Joan Crawford, for instance, was sporting a bronzed look as early as the '30s. And versions of the look Brigitte Bardot wore in the '60s—dark, smoky eyes combined with pale lips—have reappeared throughout the '90s and in recent years. The red lips and black eyeliner popular in the '50s are no longer considered retro but, rather, very elegant, as they were then. Today, the glamourizing techniques used for enhancing, accentuating, lengthening, and enlarging facial features are very similar to those that have been used throughout the century. In terms of classic drama and true glamour, there is no better example or lesson than studying the smoky eye of the '20s or the eyeliner application of Greta Garbo in the '30s. Even if you do not wish to recreate that exact look in its entirety, there are particular details of the popular styles of each decade with which you can experiment, create your own look, and have a lot of fun.

Use metallics over color to add sensual highlights. I lined the model's eyes with a vibrant blue pencil and used a turquoise cream shadow on the lid before applying a neutral shadow and then blue and gold powder shadows. I used gold shine to accent the cheeks and a pearly lip color.

twentieth-century looks

In the '20s

The makeup style of the '30s was rounded, childish, and innocent, yet strongly painted and sexual. These contradictions were epitomized by actresses such as Clara Bow, Louise Brooks, and the exotic Pola Negri.

Eyebrows were penciled or painted on in rather unusual shapes; they were well spaced and whimsical, often slightly descending or drawn straight out, giving the face a distinct expression that was important for the silent movies of this era. A faint touch of red (a color which registers well on black-and-white film and is also great for accentuating blue eyes) was often blended into a delicate shadow over the entire surface of the eyelid. A faint line was drawn under the eyes and blended to make it shadowy and indistinct and to avoid a hollow-eyed effect.

Rouge was applied to give the cheeks a rounded, doll-like look, even though in magazines women were encouraged to mix blusher colors together or with face powder to make them more natural. Women were told to first outline the cupid's bow of their upper lip in liquid rouge, drawing the lip shape they would have chosen if they could, and then apply their lipstick. Another common practice in the late '20s was to divide the upper lip into two painted halves separated by a vertical line of natural skin.

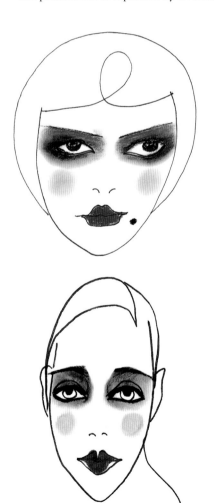

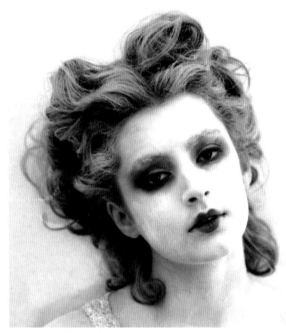

'20s-style, Mary Pickford-inspired look. Heavily shadowed eyes and small lips. *Photo by Hollister Lowe, 1996.*

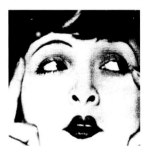

In the '30s

The stock market crash of 1929 created the worst depression America had ever seen, and people no longer felt the urge to be as wild and carefree as they did before. The face of the '30s became symmetrical, sculpted, and sensuous. Max Factor, a makeup artist for MGM movie studios, invented pancake makeup, the first water-soluble cake foundation. Before long, women everywhere wore uniformly flat, chalky, beige-to-tan complexions, often with a clear line of demarcation around their necks.

People in America and elsewhere sought to escape the problems of the everyday world through the American cinema. Hollywood and the films of such studios as MGM dominated Western culture. Inspiration came from such movie stars like the legendary Swedish-American actress Greta Garbo. Perfection was the key word to describe the look of the '30s: eyes were still strong but not as shadowed as they had been in the '20s, and lined with very heavy false lashes. The crease of the eye was accentuated. Brows grew higher and higher, and women began wearing custom-blended foundations and powders that matched their skin tones and hid imperfections. Lips were glorified by a definite, sharp, clear outline that followed the natural line of the lips more closely, using a fine sable brush and a particular kind of very concentrated cream color. This technique made for real cinema lips: perfectly shaped and beautifully colored. The makeup styles of the silver screen made lip gloss mainstream, and popular lip colors were subdued browns, ivories, creams, and roses. Bright lipsticks like red and pink were worn only sparingly. Shades were chosen to complement the wearer's natural coloring.

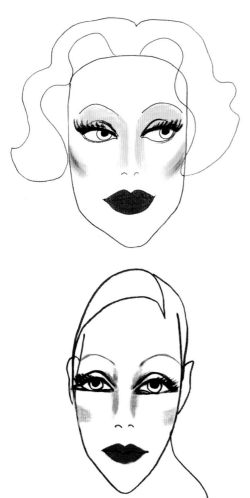

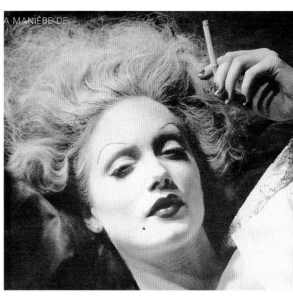

'30s-style, Jean Harlow-inspired look. I hid the brow with nose putty and base, then drew in thin brows. I applied false eyelashes and gave her large, defined lips—a departure from the style of the '20s.
Photo by Claus Wickrath.

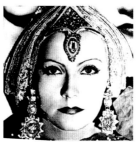

In the '40s

With the advent of World War II and America's escape from the Great Depression, makeup styles again changed. Sophisticated perfection was still popular. In general, however, in the '40s there was a trend towards a softer, sweeter, more girlish look than in the preceding decade; makeup emphasized the lips rather than the eyes. The "face" of the war relief effort was wholesome and approachable, with a façade of simplicity and gentility. The importance of a flawless complexion was emphasized, and women wore both base and powder. Max Factor made the colored pancake makeup he used for cinema makeup in colors more suitable for the women to wear on the street. Women were encouraged to apply foundation with a "feather" touch as a light base to "hold" powder, not drown the complexion. Eyes were made up with subtlety. Often, no eyeshadow or eyeliner was worn; if it was, the shadow was a soft fawn or light skin tone color, and the liner was much lighter than the dark colors of the '30s. Lashes changed dramatically from the '30s, and they were usually only lightly coated with mascara rather than heavily accentuated. Brows were kept more natural looking, moderately full and arched, and occasionally filled in with a matching color pencil. Rouge styles were somewhat of a hybrid of the '20s and '30s looks: somewhat rounded and unstructured, yet recognizing the natural contours of the cheekbone. Warm pink was the most common color choice. Lips were lined, enlarged, and rounded. Women were advised by *Vogue* magazine to define and draw them in using a brush with two shades of lipstick. In the '40s, there was a larger variety of lip colors than ever before. Towards the end of the decade, lip colors were cherry red and were applied by following the natural lip line.

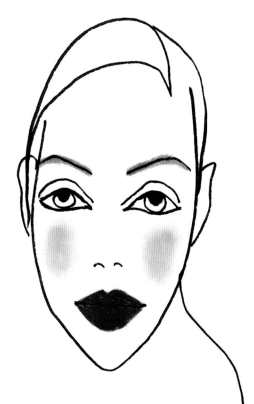

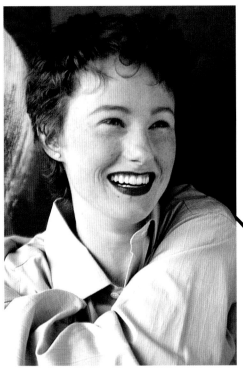

Nude lid, stronger brow, and larger lips.

In the '50s

In the U.S. post war period of the '50s, the haute couture French designer influence was strong, and makeup trends reflected that polish and elegance. The winter of 1949–50 in Paris saw the beginning a revolution in eye makeup that caught on all over: the doe-eyed look. Foundations were pale, with no trace of pink. Lip colors were darker, and rouge was not worn as much. Cake-powder compacts were back. The cosmetics market was flooded with mascara, eyeshadow, and lining pencils. Eyes were lined with black as well as colored pencils, upper eyelids were shadowed, eyebrows were penciled, and lashes were darkened with mascara. New lipstick shades were now being brought out twice a year, and shorter hairdos were fashionable. An exaggerated version of this look, called the Mandarin makeup, also originated in Paris, but its influence spread mainly through the shaping of the brows.

The outer ends of the eyebrows were entirely plucked out, and new brows penciled in a great upward and outward sweep. The beginning part of the brows was thickened, and the eyelids were shaded in white up to the brows. The eyes were lined with an upwards sweep in the outer corners, following the line of the brows. A style made popular by that fabulously sexy French movie star Brigitte Bardot at the end of the '50s was the ever-enduring dark smokey eye/pale-lipped look, which was then perfected in the '60s (see section on "The Smoky Eye").

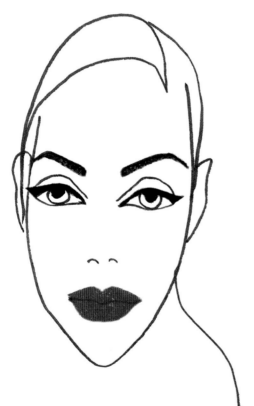

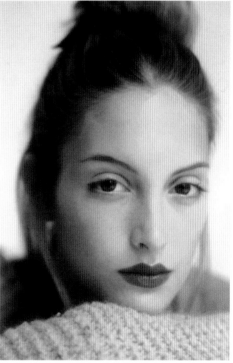

Eyes were lined with black, lip colors were darker. *Photo by Elisabeth Novick for* Grazia, *1992.*

In the '60s

By 1963, the doe-eyed look was out. Again, "eye shapes" started changing and becoming rounder. Tanning, which had disappeared in the '50s, was never more popular, and faces became contoured and highlighted with shine. Makeup again emphasized the eyes, making them very large, and no longer gave so much focus to the mouth. Eyeliner, now brown or gray rather than black, was applied so that it thickened a bit in the center of the lashline and stopped at the end of the eye. The crease line from styles popular in the 30s reappeared, giving the eye a rounder effect. Lip colors became very pale. Mascaras were made in a large variety of colors and formulas to lengthen the lashes.

By 1964, a sculptured style of blush was getting underway. Loads of tawny makeup blusher was applied around the face, hairline, jawbone, and chin. Gold shades were popular, even in the daytime, and contrasting makeup with one's clothes was in. Adults were no longer the only users of cosmetics: The teenage market had skyrocketed. A survey of teens around the mid-60s indicated that two thirds in America had worn lipstick.

Shine was also all the rage. In 1969, British *Vogue* wrote, "First a new face—clear and shining . . . Color your lips with natural shiny stain . . . Your eyes must look wide awake and shiny." Eyebrows were very plucked and thin. False eyelashes were at first thick and short, but were replaced by much longer lashes spaced farther apart. Then brows became thinner and more rounded. The crease of the eyes was accentuated, and the liner took a downward tilt; lids were lightly colored in light, grayish shades. Eyelashes, which were drawn in under the lower lashes at the beginning of the decade, were being applied individually to the base of both the upper and lower lashes by the end of the '60s.

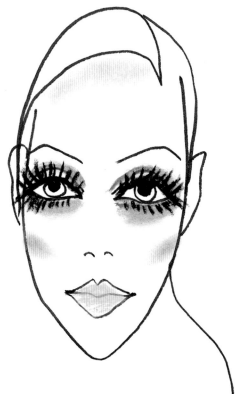

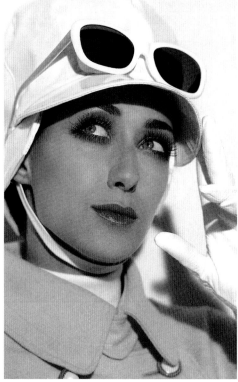

Long false eyelashes and glossy lips.
Photo by Walter Chin for German Vogue, *1992.*

In the '70s

In the '70s, television had a worldwide impact and was replacing the influence of movies on makeup and hairstyles. The program *Charlie's Angels* sparked a trend that was a mixture of styles of the '60s and '70s, and that trend continued on into the '80s. The look combined the tanned, shiny face of the '60s with a more elongated eye makeup, a pale, pearlized lip color, and blue pencil-liner in the inner rim of the lower eyelid and under the eyes.

In America, as in England, permissiveness in makeup hit a new peak for a short while in 1970. Rainbows were painted around the eyes, lashes were reddened, and eyebrows were painted green. The photographer Sarah Moon brought back the pale-faced, doll-lipped look with enormously large, dark, painted, round, smokey, '20s-style eyes for the fashions of the designer Biba, who was all the rage in England. In addition to fashion, Biba had a wonderful array of makeup colors in painting palettes. Purple nail polish, mahogany lipstick, black face gloss, prune watercolors, and yellow foundation. Mary Quant (who had her own line of cosmetics) also sold makeup crayons in all colors.

Towards the middle of the '70s, the style changed. The extreme was very made up, pale, matte faces with strong, very visible blush applied on a diagonal under the cheekbones. Strong, elongated eyes were shadowed with harsh, very metallic shades of violet, orange, and pink. Shadow was applied under the eyes, and colored or black pencil almost always lined the inner rim of the lower eye. Brows were still undeveloped, and lips were colored with strong fuchsia and very glossy reds, which became more matte towards the end of the decade.

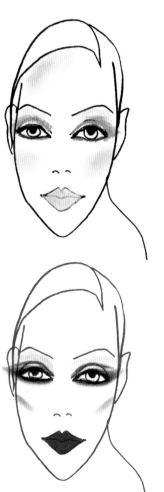

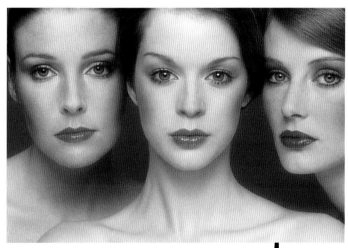

Pale matte faces with visible blush, thin brows, and color and shine in the eye shadow.
Photo by Jacques Rouchon for Helene Curtis.

In the '80s

At the beginning of the '80s, all the designers had different makeup styles. They ranged from the glamorous look of Thierry Mugler to the innovative splashes of color I was doing for Rei Kawakubo of Comme des Garcons. However, a strong trend throughout the decade was the pale, matte face with strong, grey taupe shadows on the eyes and a strong, red, glossy lip.

Towards the end of the '80s, the matte lip colors that had been shown in Paris at the end of the '70s were becoming popular in the United States. Red lipstick became more and more matte. Base and foundation became more "nude," and lips were more brown and matte. Eyes, too, became browner and smokier, and the most important aspect of the makeup in the '80s was eyebrow: It was for the most part unplucked and made to look thick, unless you had naturally thick brows like Brooke Shields.

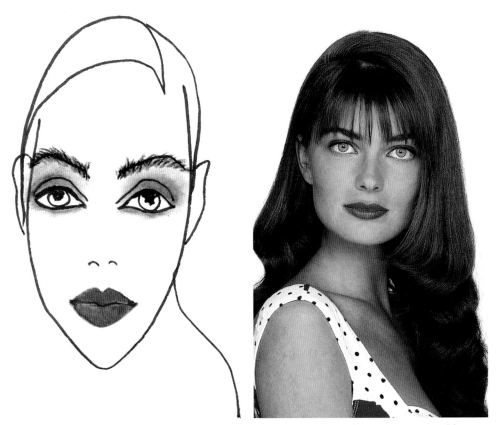

Thick brows, a pale face, and strong red lips.
Photo by Jacques Malignon.

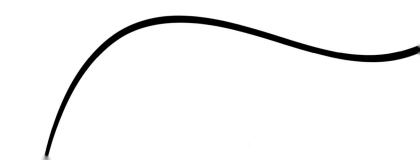

In the '90s

In the beginning to mid '90s, glamour was back with a vengeance. No one wanted color, and everything was very matte and brown. There were spurts of discrete color, such as the dark ruby-red lipstick made popular by Norma Kamali and in Francis Ford Coppola's 1992 movie *Dracula*. In the beginning of the '90s, however, a very matte, finished look was back, with monochromatic brown shading on the eyes. Compact powder foundation was applied to the face, giving a smooth, even finish, often applied over another base to give more coverage and uniformity. Makeup was done in the traditional manner, with each classic step completed. Liner was kept close to the eye, and lids were fairly light, especially under the brow on the brow bone. Lips were well defined, enlarged, and heavily lined with pencil; lipsticks were either beige, brown, or burgundy, which was a look promoted by celebrity makeup artist Kevin Aucoin. Everything was perfected, taken to an extreme. Lips were enlarged by any means possible, and brows clipped and waxed into perfectly tailored shapes.

Towards the middle of the '90s, lids became much more lightly colored with soft pearl shades; they were also either discretely lined or not lined at all; lips became more strong, deep, matte ruby shades and more brown than the vampire-red rub—more burgundy, but still very lined. A natural, transparent, understated look also came in at the mid '90s, running parallel to the more sophisticated, dark-lipped/pale eye. This understated look has shown up in every decade; this time it was cleaner and more finished.

Heavy matte lipcolors became more shiny and glittery in the late '90s, perhaps to contradict the very natural look in vogue at the same time. Glitter was first used on the lips, then it spread to the rest of the face, the cheeks, and eyes. In the late '90s, women wanted to experiment again. The shiny-skinned look that had appeared briefly in the '80s came back with a vengeance. Everyone glistened and seemed almost sweaty (at least in photos). Piercing ears, tongues, and noses became fashionable, as did tattooing.

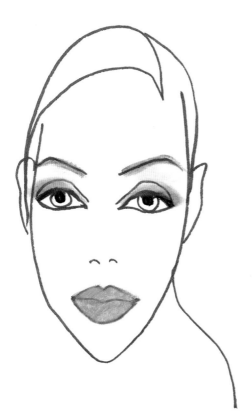
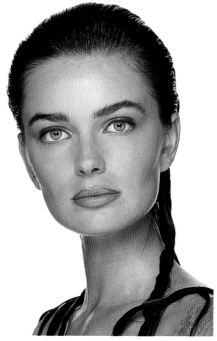

Matte lip color and a shiny-skinned look.
Photo by Jacques Malignon.

period pointers

Perfectly Powdered

Since as far back as the '20s, colored face powders have been popular. If someone were naturally dark, such as someone with an olive complexion, they wore ocher or cream powder to brighten their skin, and fair blondes were encouraged to wear mauve powder to give the skin a clear, delicate look or even dead-white powder for a more bizarre effect. In the '70s, I worked a lot with colored powders during the fashion shows to strengthen the individuality of each model, often using mauve to make the models look whiter under the strong lights. Today, there are some beautiful, lightweight colored powders that are great to use all over or just to give certain parts of the face matte accents. Lilac powders tend to accentuate paleness; they lighten and whiten skin. Banana shades, depending on their depth of color, can lighten and brighten ivory (fair skin with a yellowish undertone) and deeper yellow-toned skins. Peach shades are good if you want to add warmth rather than brightness to yellow-toned skins; deeper shades of peach powder are great for adding a warm glow to most African-American skin tones, although they do not look good on the deeper blue skin tones, which look best with a cooler shade of dark brown powder which better enhances the natural coloring of this skin.

A light dusting of powder over concealer actually brings out a radiant complexion and gives a fresh-faced look.
Photo by Elisabeth Novick for Grazia, 1992.

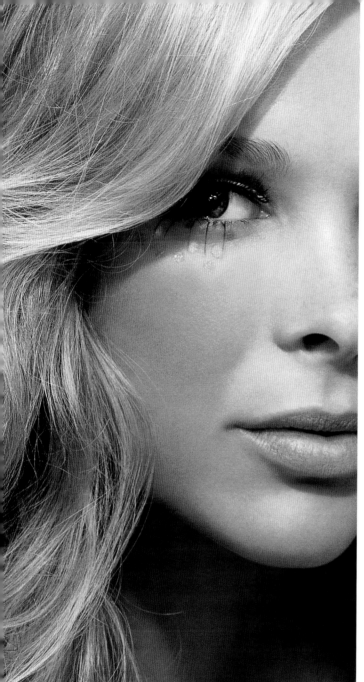

A Fashionable Tan

Tanned skin has been fashionable since the 30s; it was prompted by Coco Chanel in France and popularized by Joan Crawford in America in her movie *This Modern Age*. As early as 1919, the American magazine *Delineator's* beauty columnist Celia Caroline Cole observed, "A nice, comfortable, careless tan is what every woman ought to have in the summer if she wants to help her skin all she can." Obviously, we know better now. *Exposure to the sun can cause wrinkles and other kinds of skin damage, not to mention skin cancer.* As early as the '30s, however, companies offered products that simulated the sun-kissed look, such as tanning lotions, creams, and body makeup. You didn't have to bake in the sun to look tanned. Bronzers began appearing on the market, and people everywhere embraced this new chic. Today's self-tanners are much more sophisticated and no longer give you an artificial, orangey look. They allow you to simulate a tan, which you can further enhance by wearing warm-toned gel and cream bronzers on your cheekbones and any other place the sun would normally highlight. Don't overdo it with bronzer: wearing too much of it can have the opposite effect by drowning your features and dulling your face rather than brightening it.

A cream base with lots of warm blush and powder. A strong green eyeshadow at the base of the upper lashes and green eyelashes. '60s retro: thin lashes and dots drawn under the eyes. Pale pink lip color.

Photo by Michael Myers for YM magazine, 2001.

The Tamed Brow

You don't need to wear heavy makeup to glamourize your look, but you do need to tame your brows! Well-spaced and whimsical in the '20s, high and arched in the '30s, thick and exotic as per Thierry Mugler in late '70s — glamourous brows were glamourous because they were tamed. Today, brows are cut, waxed above and below, tweezed, and tattooed. Waxing and tattooing should be done by a professional. Before you try such a drastic step, if you have thick brows, try taming them by playing around with soap. Soften a bar of soap with water, rub your eyebrow brush on the soap, the brush your brows with the soap until you have enough soap on them to flatten them with your fingertip. Then cover them as best you can with a cream concealer or base and powder over the cream with a transparent powder to make them flesh toned. The brows will not be perfectly hidden, but enough for you to see how you would look with a different shaped brow once you pencil on a new brow. If are considering tattooing your brows, make sure you understand that tattooing is permanent! Eyebrow shapes go out of fashion, so be very sure you are ready to commit to wearing the particular style and placement you choose *forever*. Discuss it with your tattooist. No matter what your coloring is, I recommend that if you tattoo your brows, you go no deeper than a very neutral shade of brown. Then you can always deepen the color with pencil if you like; black is very artificial and can look harsh. If you tattoo your brows black, you have no options for softening them.

Apply jewels to the brows with false-eyelash glue. *Photo Art Kane for Italian* Vogue, *1986.*

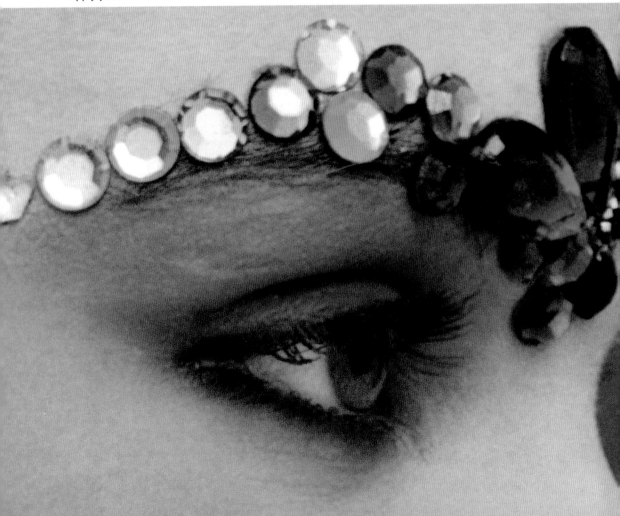

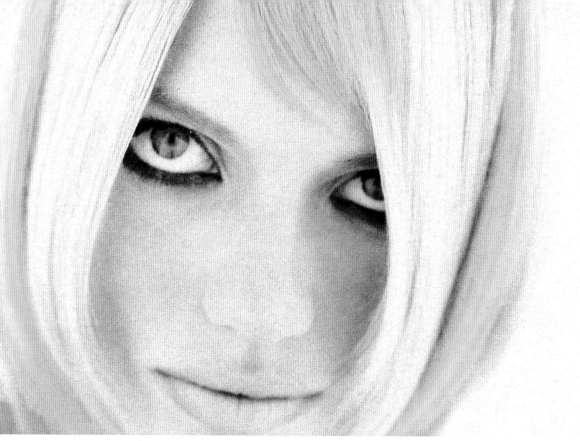

Heavy under-eye liner with a heavy lid can create a sultry look. *Photo by Diego Uchitel, 1995. Hair: John Sahag.*

The Sultry Eye

In the '30s, the makeup Greta Garbo wore in her screen appearances was concentrated heavily on her eyes. Unusual and elaborate, it was an adaptation of stage makeup whose goal was to enlarge an actor's eyes so the audience could see them better. To recreate Garbo's big, glamourous eye makeup, first accentuate the heaviness of your lid by applying a white or very light color cream or powder eye shadow to the mobile part of the lid next to the eye. Depending on how high you blend the shading over the pupil, when you blend the "crease outline," you can dramatically alter the shape of the eye. If you would like to make the eyes look less downward sloping, make sure you do not blend the color out onto the brow bone above the pupil. Garbo's black liner extended downwards from the base of the upper lashes to join with the extended crease line, forming a triangle which extended the size and shape of the eyes. You can replace the black liner with brown for a softer effect. Garbo then applied a few false eyelashes to the outer corner of the upper lid of her eyes.

In the '50s, Marilyn Monroe wore a different kind of sultry eye makeup; hers was a rather unusual method of lining that winged upwards in the outer corner—it was thicker in the inner corner of the eye and narrow in the outer corner, and then it turned up, creating a sultry, almost sleepy look.

The Doe Eye

Starting on the runway models of Christian Dior and popularized by actresses such as Audrey Hepburn, the winter of 1949–50 heralded the beginning of a revolution in eye makeup in Paris: the doe-eyed look. The eyes were lined with a black pencil, cake, or liquid eyeliner and lengthened with an upwards slope at the outer corners.

To do this, apply your eyeliner the same way you normally would, by beginning the line in the outer, upper corner of your lid along the lash line, making the line thickest at the outer corner and thinner as you approach the inner corner. To achieve a doe eye, extend a small line from just above the outer corner of the eye, winging it outwards and upwards so it extends beyond the outer edge of the lash line by about a quarter on an inch. How far out and up you should extend the line depends on how strong a shape you want to give your eye. Join the end of the small extension to the eyeliner at the base of the lashes and fill in the space formed. Always look at yourself straight ahead in the mirror to see the effect you are creating with your eyeliner. Each of your eyes is different, and you may need to draw the liner on one thicker than on the other to balance the eye and rather than accentuate their difference.

A colorful doe eye. Apply a shimmery pink over the entire lid, define the crease and under eye with an orange eye shadow. For the liner, draw a short line from just above the outer corner of the eye. At the center, join the outer corner of the line with the line at the base of the lashes, then fill in any space. *Photo by Bruno Gaget.*

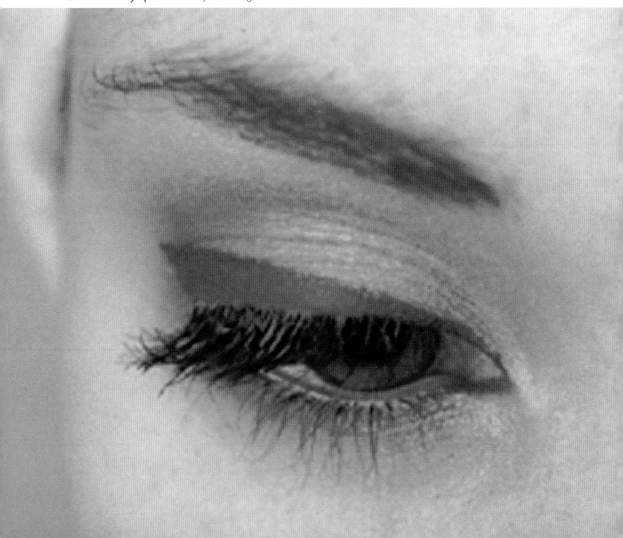

The Cat Eye

This eye was popular in the '70s. Begin by applying pencil inside the lower rim of the eye, then blend shadow under the eye and extend it to lengthen the eye. It is very important to keep the area of the brow bone light. Darken around the eye, especially in the outer corner. Blend the dark shading outwards, and just keep adding until you achieve the intensity you are looking for.

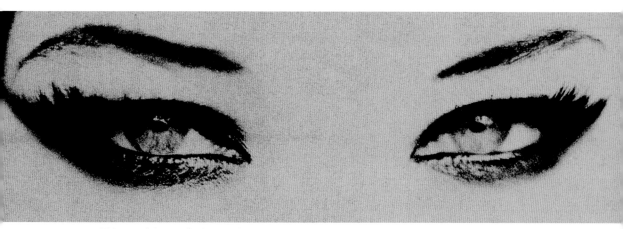

Add heavy false eyelashes to the outer corners of the upper lids after finishing the cat eye to make it wing upwards even more.

In the '50s, Marilyn Monroe lengthened and lined her sultry eyes by applying her liner in an unusual way. She thickened the liner slightly in the inner corner, going thinner over the outer part of the upper lid, then winging the liner upwards from the outer corner of the eyes. A small white line was applied under the wing of the liner to accentuate it and another touch of white was applied to the center of the lid just above the liner.

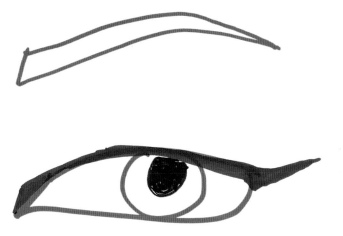

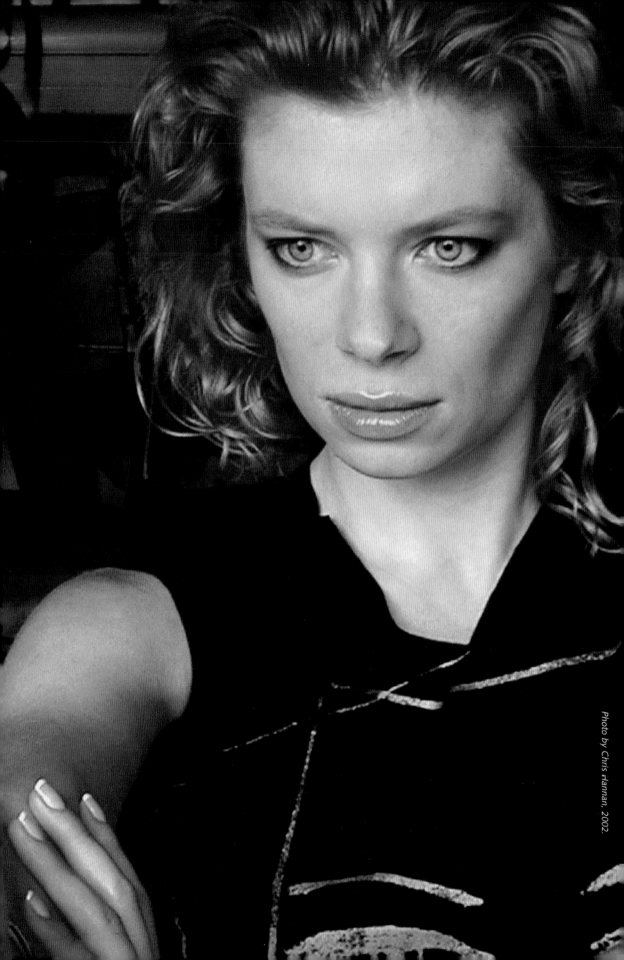

The Smoky Eye

Ever since Brigitte Bardot's smoky eyes took the late '50s and early '60s by storm, there have been many versions of this style which are still very popular today (it's one of my daughter Daisy's favorites). Makeup masters such as Way Bandy in the '70s and Kevin Aucoin in the '90s built their fortunes and fame perfecting this look. In fact, I myself have been asked to do a neutral smoky eye more than any other style—believe me, there is no makeup more difficult to do well. Before trying to do this style of eye makeup, go back and reread the section on eyes in Chapter 2, "The Basics." Take note of the tips on keeping the inner corners of your eye light if you have close-set eyes.

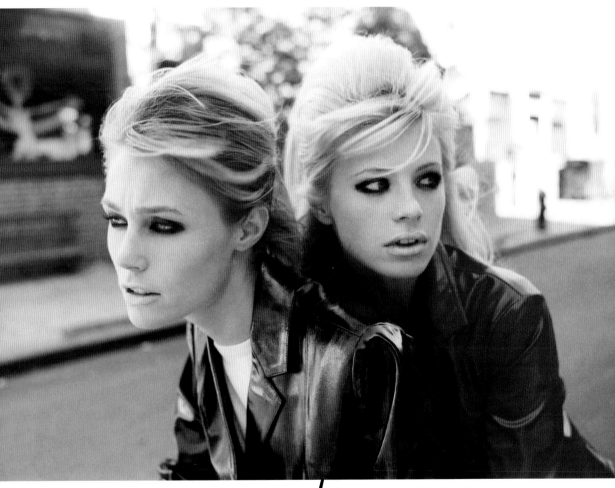

A '90s version of the Bardot smoky eye for *Amica* magazine.
Photo Alessandro D'Andrea, 1995. Styling: Cinzia Brandi.

How to Do the Smoky Eye

A smoky eye is best realized with matte shadows, then pearlized ones to give highlights. There are various ways of realizing different intensities of this eye makeup.

You can also do any of these steps using a color other than deep brown or black. You can get a smoky eye using deep shades of blue, green, or violet.

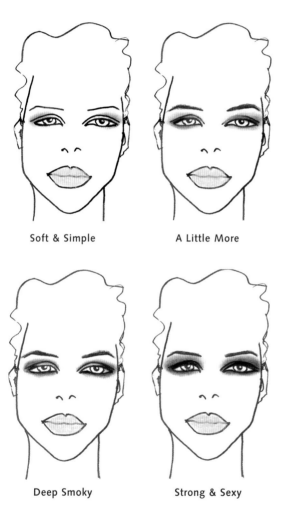

Soft & Simple

A Little More

Deep Smoky

Strong & Sexy

Soft & Simple For a *soft & simple* version, use only one shade of shadow. Rim the eyes with a gray or black pencil or gray shadow. Apply it to the very base of the lashes all around the eye, making sure the color is more intense at the upper, outer corner. Blend the color outwards and upwards, just past the crease.

A Little More For a *little more intensity*, use two shadows. Blend your first shade, which should be gray or brown of medium intensity, from the base of the lashes outwards and upwards on the lid. Apply a little under the eye at the very base of the lower lashes. Now take a deeper, more intense shade of gray or brown and blend it with a brush over the first color in the upper, outer corner of the eyes, at the very base of the eyelashes.

Deep Smoky To achieve a *deep smoky look*, use three shadows. Apply a deep shade in the crease of the eye, under the eye, and in the outer, upper corner of the eye. Blend the shadow outwards and over the brow bone slightly; also blend under the eye. Apply black to the very base of the lower lashes at the outer corner. Apply a light powder on the brow bone (ivory or white). Apply a black or very dark pencil to the inner rim of the lower lashes.

Strong & Sexy For a *dramatically strong and sexy look*, use four shadows. Follow the instructions for creating the "deep smoky eye." Next, put a shade of medium intensity on a large-headed eye shadow brush and sweep the color over the entire eyelid, up to the brows. Take your black pencil and line the eyes from the very inner corner to the outer corner, making the line heavier in the outer corner. Blend the pencil and press black eye shadow powder into it with the tip of a brush (the mixture of the powder over the creamier pencil will make the color stronger).

Neutral smoky layers

Each layer can be worn individually or in combination with the others to create a strong smoky eye.

1. Blend a soft taupe shade of demi pearl shadow over your eyelid shadow to the very base of the upper lashes. This will create a base to make blending the deeper shades easier.

2. Blend a deeper shade of grey under the base of the lower lashes and on the outer half of the upper lid to just past the crease of the eye.

3. Blend dark brown shadow around the eye at the base of both the upper and lower lashes. Blend the shadow outwards.

4. Line the lashes with a black pencil over and under the eyes. Draw the line thinner in the inner corner and over the pupil, then thicker in the outer third of the eyes. Soften and blend the line outwards with an eyeliner brush. Powder on top of the pencil with transluscent powder with a pressing motion of a clean eyeshadow brush. Then blend a black powder by pressing it carefully with a small brush onto the area where the black pencil was applied.

5. All the steps combined.

To make this makeup even more intense, draw a line of black liquid or cake eyeliner into the very base of the lashes.

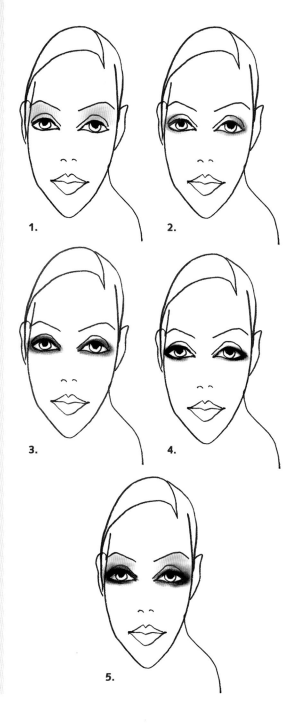

Small adjustments make an incredible difference in adapting a makeup to a particular woman's face or style. If you're fifty years old and you still want to wear dark eye shadow, and heavy eye makeup and eyelashes, wear them. But update and adjust your makeup by swiping a Q-tip under the eyes across your makeup, define your brows more, and soften your cheek color and the line of your lips. Otherwise, such a strong makeup can look overly harsh and accentuate the lines and creases in an older woman's face. If you are Asian or if you have heavy eyelids, apply more makeup under the eye to give the shape of your eyes balance and to avoid making them look "top heavy."

Fluttering False Eyelashes

In the '20s, after World War I, makeup styles reflected a spirit of liberty and vivaciousness—women felt free to experiment and were unafraid of sending "mixed" signals about who they were through what they wore. Cosmetics started to be seen as tools of expression and as fun accessories. Lashes were tinted and sometimes even beaded. Beading the lashes involved putting a wax-like substance on the end of each separate eyelash, often with a matchstick, thus creating a beaded effect. In the '30s, women wore false eyelashes of bewildering length or used "eyelash irons" (the predecessors of today's eyelash curlers) to curl their own.

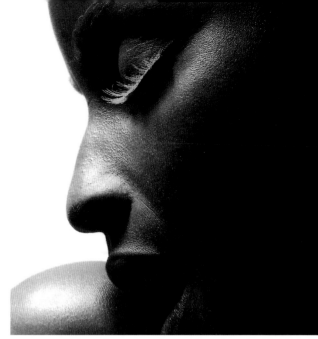

Bands of real-hair false eyelashes.
Photo by Bruno Gaget for Zoozoom.com, 2001.

To apply individual lashes or clusters of lashes:

1. Hold each one with tweezers.
2. Dip the base lightly into the eyelash glue (which usually comes with the lashes you buy—the best glue is white because it becomes transparent).
3. With the lash poised so that it will be curling "up" when in place, press the base with the glue carefully between your real lashes into the very base of your lash line.

How to apply a band of false lashes:

1. Remove the lash from the "platform" with tweezers or with your fingernails. Be sure the lash fits your own eyelid; if it doesn't, cut off the excess from the outer part of the lashes (about 1/4 cm).
2. Rim the edge of the band (remember that they should positioned so that they are curling "up" when placed) that you're going to press to the base of your real lashes with the eyelash glue.
3. Wait a few minutes until the glue is slightly tacky.
4. Apply the band to the base of the natural lashes by first pressing the center onto the base of the center of your real lashes with an orange stick, and then pressing the corners down.

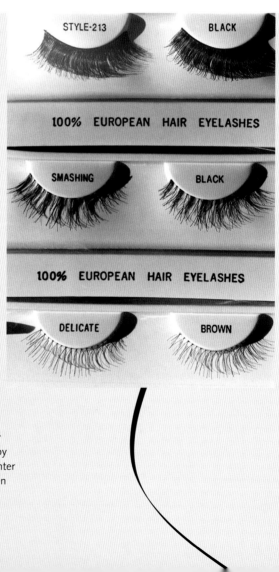

In the late '50s and early '60s, bands of thick, furry false lashes made of real hair were worn. The extremely talented Pablo Manzoni, the star of the makeup scene in New York at that time, was working for Elizabeth Arden and applying double and even triple bands of false lashes. Lashes were also *drawn in* under the eye by making thin, downward-sloping lines with a pencil or liquid liner. By the beginning of the '70s, false individual lashes were being applied to the base of both the upper and lower lash lines.

False eyelashes either come individually or in clusters, semi-bands, or full bands. The full bands range from the most natural (feathered with a light-colored base) to the most dramatic (tightly packed, thick lashes with a dark base). I recommend you apply all your other cosmetics before you apply false eyelashes so you can better judge how they enhance your eye shape.

Unless you are very dark, short brown lash clusters will look the most natural. Short ones can be applied alone. Or, to make your lashes look long, after applying two short clusters of false lashes in the outer corners of the eyes, apply three medium-length clusters, then apply two more short clusters. If you already have long lashes, you can make them look even longer. Working inwards from the outer corner of the eye, apply one short cluster, then one medium-length, then three or four long clusters, followed by one or two medium-length clusters at the inner corner. When applying lashes under the eyes, make sure to place them once again in the very base of the lashes, this time with the lashes curling down.

If you want to keep the soft effect of lightweight lashes, do not apply eyeliner over the base. However, unless you want a simple, soft look, it is usually best to cover the base of the false lashes with a thin line of eyeliner. Eyelash glue also happens to be a good way to attach any other accessory to your brows or eyelid that you may want to play with, such as beads, sequins, or glitter.

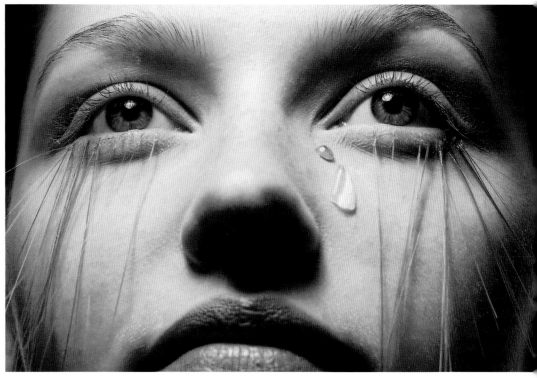

Light orange on lid, orange on crease line. False-hair lashes glued under eyes and plexiglass stones glued with the same eyelash glue under the eye. No mascara. *Photo by Bruno Gaget for Zoozoom.com, 2001.*

Contouring

Ella Adelia Fletcher gave the following advice at the beginning of the twentieth century in her book *The Woman Beautiful*: "The first touch of artificial color is given to the face to bring up the adjacent features to harmonize with one another. A startlingly white nose cuts the face in two, so a touch of rouge, deftly blended, is needed on the nostrils; if the nose be large, a very little [rouge] on the sides will lessen its prominence. The chin, and the lobes and edges of the ears, too, must be touched with rouge very delicately and in a rotary motion, which will make streaks impossible and leave no edges." Her advice is still sound today. In the '20s, rouge was used to make the face look childish and doll-like. In the '30s, rouge was used to contour and sculpt the cheekbones, making them appear higher and more prominent. By the height of the '60s, the sculpted look was once again in vogue—loads of tawny makeup blusher around the face, hairline, jawbone, and chin was all the rage.

Contouring was inspired by stage makeup. Its aim is to give a face the suggestion of a more interesting bone structure than it actually has—to tone down whatever has too much of and bring out what one needs more of. The sculpted, cinema look of the '30s (made popular again in the '60s) does not have to be obvious to be effective. In certain instances, if you choose the right products, you can make an enormous difference in the appearance of your face and neck and make them look noticeably slimmer. You can do this with contouring powders or creams in neutral brown tones. For extra depth and strength, first use a creamy product, then powder the face and apply shading with a contouring powder. (I'll explain exactly how in the next paragraph.) A contouring powder or cream must be a matte, neutral brown shade that is quite a lot deeper than your natural skin tone. Add blush after you've applied contouring to give some color. If you want to keep the overall matte effect, brush on a light or white powder to any parts of the face you would like to highlight; if you want to add a little shine, use an iridescent highlighter.

Contouring

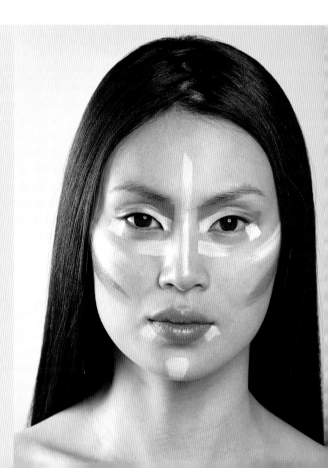

1. Sometimes white highlighter alone can be sufficient to attract the light and give the face more contouring.

2. White or a touch of a lighter concealer applied at the outer corners of the eye and the lips will give a slight lift to the general aspect of the face.

3. Highlighting on the nose will make a wide nose seem narrower.

4. The contouring under the cheekbone should not be too low, just on the underside of the bone.

5. Contouring under the jawbone will define the jawbone and slim down the neck.

Photos (both pages) by Bruno Gaget.
Hair: Mayumi for John Sahag.

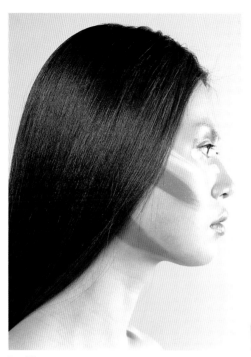

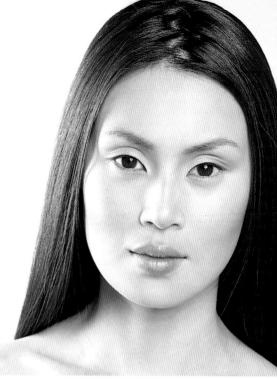

Profile.

Minami with contouring blended.

To give a full face with no visible cheekbones a more sculpted, thinner look, blend a little cream base four or five shades darker than your skin tone on the underside of the bone. Massage your face with your fingertips to find the cheekbone, and place the darker shade on the lower part of the bone. Blend it inwards towards the area just under the nose and slightly downward into the hollow of your cheeks (or where the hollow is supposed to be) with your fingertips or a dampened sponge. Take care not to apply too much in the hollow or to go too near the nose (which would make the effect harsher and very artificial). Your cheekbones and your jawbones are easy to find this way. Many women lack definition between the face and neck; blending the same deeper shade of cream base down from around the underside of the jawbone with a damp sponge (or even just using a neutral brown powder blush in this area after you have finished your makeup), will have that same slimming effect, as will lightening the jawbone. Blend your blush with the cream contouring, or brush it on after powdering.

In general, I discourage using this method to slim the nose because you can actually end up making it look fatter. I recommend highlighting the center of a wide nose (as opposed to shading the sides) to give the impression of more depth to the sides of the nose. For a professional, it is useful to know that a wide nose often goes with wide-set eyes, and the skin at the beginning of the brows on the brow bone should also probably be shaded with the same contouring powder you have chosen for the nose. The shading should just be done on the sides of the tip if the nose is concave, and very slightly in a fairly straight line (not too thick) down each side of the nose if it is straight and flat.

The parts of the face you may want to accent are the cheekbones, the forehead (if it is small), and the chin (if it is small). To make a wide or large nose look narrower, highlight the center of the nose as opposed to shading the sides, which is difficult to do naturally. Many women lack definition between the face and the neck; you can achieve this by lightening the jawbone and deepening the color of the neck area just under the jaw bone to make the face "pop out" more. Blend your blush in with the cream contouring, or blush it on after powdering.

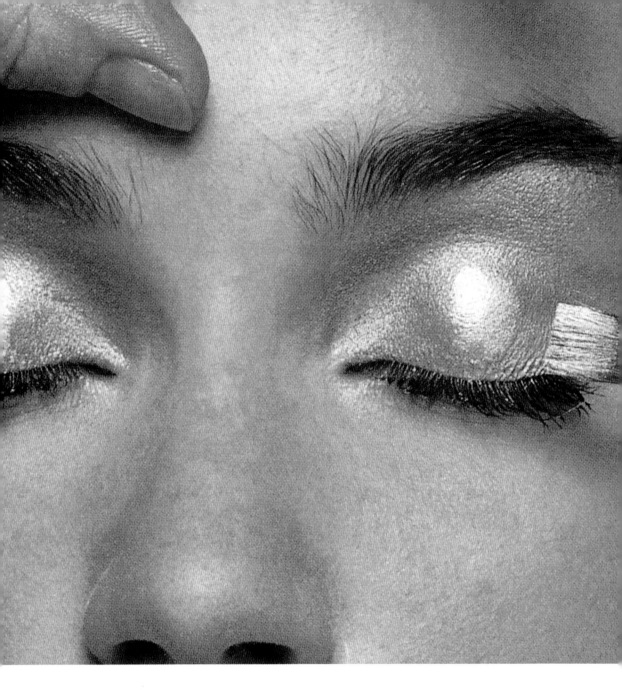

Magnetic Metallics

In the world of makeup, the popularity of shine fluctuates. Whenever it comes back into fashion, it does so in a way that's slightly different from its last incarnation. If you have clear skin with a pure, ivory/yellow undertone, a touch of antique gold will always look beautiful on you. If you don't like the way you look in blush, a touch of gold shine looks great on its own as a natural highlighter on the cheekbones. It also gives a stronger accent to the cheekbones if you apply it over your blush. Gold also looks wonderful on deeper, olive-toned skins. Bronze also adds warmth and shine to tan or darker skin, and white pearlescent cream or powder can either accentuate the opalescence of pale skin or give lighter accents to dark skin. Heavy metallic cosmetics rarely look good all over the face, but if you have great skin and bone structure, you can mix a little with a touch of Vaseline and smooth it on your face for all-over shine.

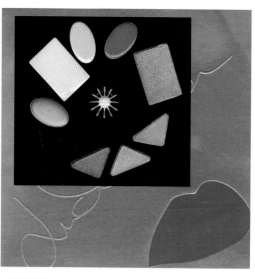

Metallic color palette.

One gold brush stroke. To do this, wet a one-inch-wide, fairly stiff paintbrush and rub it on an iridescent blush or pearl eyeshadow, then paint a stroke down your face. *Photo by Hans Feurer for French* ELLE*. Model: Cecilia Chancellor.*

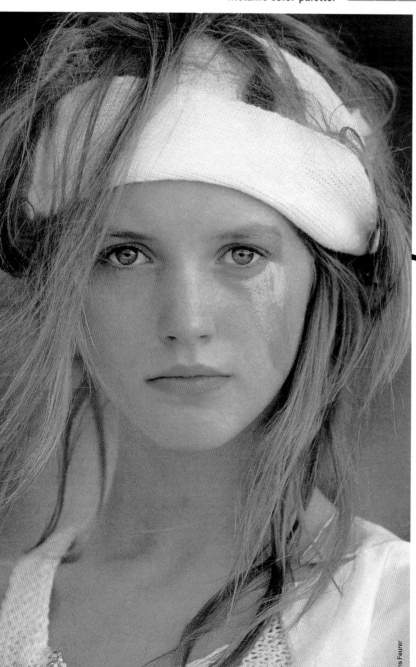

Hans Feurer

Luscious Lips

In the '20s, when coloring the lips was definitely in. According to Richard Corson's book *Fashions in Makeup*, magazines told women to "apply color with the finger, following the contour of the lips, but stopping short of the corners. Accent the curve of the upper lip, but put little if any color on the lower lip, as it [will] get sufficient color from the one above." Women were told to first outline their Cupid's bow in liquid rouge, drawing the shape they would have chosen if they could, and then to apply their lipstick.

Many people wrongly believe that dark lip colors make lips look smaller. Small, deftly defined lips with a bright or a dark color can look bigger. If you have very narrow lips and wish to make your mouth more voluptuous, it is almost easier to do it with a deeper matte lip color than it is with a more soft one. Begin by applying your lip color normally, then take a lip brush or a pencil in the same shade as your lip color and start applying color from the center of both the upper and lower lip outward. Lips often have a stronger edge slightly inside of an fainter, outer one; to make the lips look fuller, gently use the lip brush to blend the lip color to that fainter *outer edge*. Be careful not to apply the color too heavily on the lower, outer corners of the lips because this will bring the mouth down. Always begin by defining the center of the lips with the brush, then rolling the color and going over the darker edge in the center first if necessary. If your lips are thicker in the center and narrower on the sides, you should define the center first and then go over the darker edges to balance them out, working gradually outwards around the lips. To make this type of lip softer, dot a light shade of lip color on the center. Another trick to enlarge the lips is to brush a light line of iridescent or metallic powder around the lip line after you have applied your lipstick; gold works well on deeper skin tones, and pearl is best on very pale ones. Blend the line into the lip color to soften it and to give it a more natural effect.

Pearly lip color attracts the light and can make lips appear larger, but this is only true for lips that are already fairly full. A very pale lip color on its own on medium-to-full lips will have a tendency to accentuate their fullness; thin lips will need more definition.

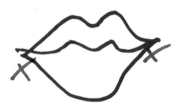

Don't go too heavy with color in the lower corners of the lips because that brings the mouth down and makes it look droopy.

Always begin lip color application by using a brush in the center of the lips and working the color outwards to define or enlarge the lips. Brace your elbow on a table to steady your hand.

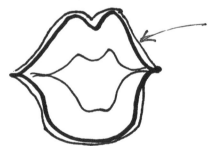

To make lips look fuller, apply your pencil or lip color right to the lighter edge of the lips.

OPPOSITE PAGE **Lips don't need to be heavily lined to be well defined—a rich color applied with a lip brush gives a full look.** *Photo by Roberto Edwards for* Paula *magazine.*

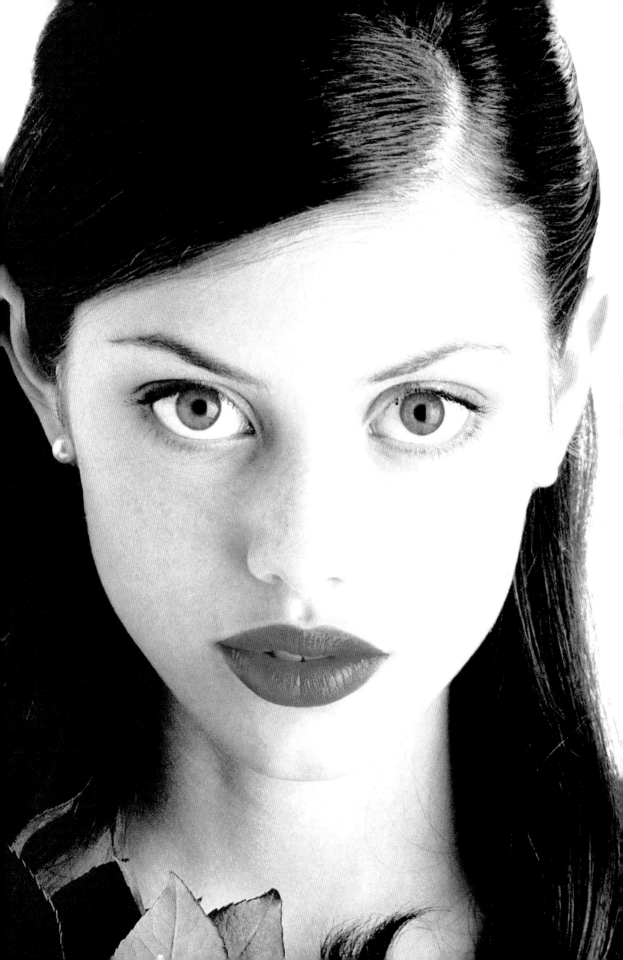

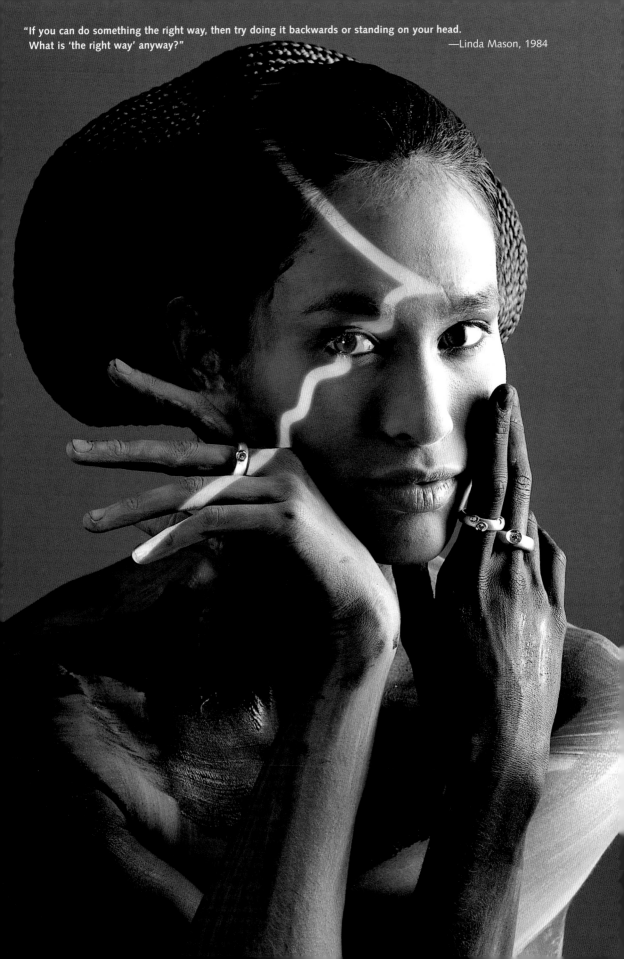

"If you can do something the right way, then try doing it backwards or standing on your head. What is 'the right way' anyway?"

—Linda Mason, 1984

CHAPTER 4

freestyle makeup

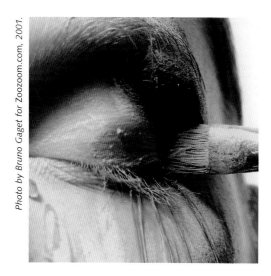

Photo by Bruno Gaget for Zoozoom.com, 2001.

Freestyle makeup represents the opposite of the glamourizing makeup techniques I demonstrated in the last chapter. Those techniques enhance facial features in a conventional manner and stay within certain parameters of color and positioning. With freestyle makeup, colors are splashed around the face like accessories, and color acts to accentuate feeling, mood, or personality, or to capture flashes of light.

During my career as a makeup artist for prêt-à-porter runway shows in Paris, I became inspired by the way fashion designers like Jean Paul Gaultier, Yohji Yamamoto, and John Galliano adopted a liberated approach to materials and structure. Their designs, along with painters like Degas and van Dongen, influenced my approach to makeup: I began to splash color around the face, stroke it on, leave it messy, smudge it, or make it more spontaneous. How does this method translate to you? First of all, with this approach, you no longer look at your face and say things like, "I would like to have bigger eyes and larger lips." You are deconstructing the way you normally see your face and looking at it like a live painting on which you are working, mixing textures and using contrasting colors.

I am not necessarily telling you to paint yourself with paintbrushes as I have done in many of these photos, although that is lots of fun. What I am saying is that a flat, almost imperceptible hint of green on your eyelids or across your face can do as much for your beauty as spending hours trying to create a smoky eye. And if do want the look of a smoky eye, then a messy, asymmetrical one with a swipe of highlighting color can be just as sexy, if not more so, than a perfect one.

Think about the way sunlight can make a beautiful pattern on your face; you can recreate that with shimmer. Each of your brows is different. Forget about symmetry and trying to make them perfect—do something as simple as brushing a different cream-color into each brow. You can really try anything. The great thing about makeup is that you can always wash it off. Freestyle makeup is just that: freeing.

Aqua and violet face and body paint intensify this model's exotic features. *Photo by Helmut Hoffmann. Model: Debbie. Art Direction: Martina Ibbels. Hair: Charles Olivier.*

what is freestyle?

Makeup is learned primarily through observation. Therefore, you can find tremendous inspiration by looking at ancient and modern art along with books, magazines, and movies. The ideas you can get from interesting people you see on the street are not as obvious, but they are just as rich. Even the oddest things can be an inspiration.

There is no strict definition of freestyle makeup. That's the beauty of it—it's anything but strict. Freestyle can be subtle: Apply a little bit of blue to each eye, or apply colors asymmetrically, and then blend them. Freestyle can be simple: Just draw a line of white or a dot of black under each eye.

You can do freestyle techniques without applying any other conventional makeup such as base, powder, or blush, or you can apply it over a conventional makeup. It is much easier to adjust and change if you do it without conventional makeup, but if your skin tone is uneven, you may be more comfortable using a little base to even it slightly.

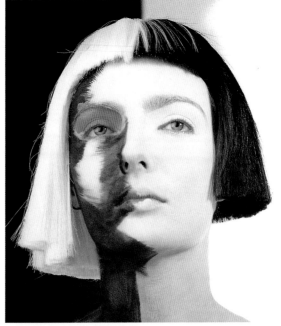

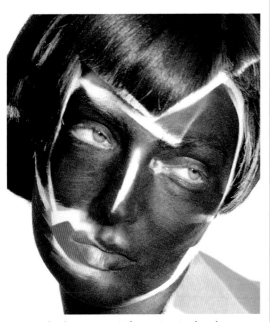

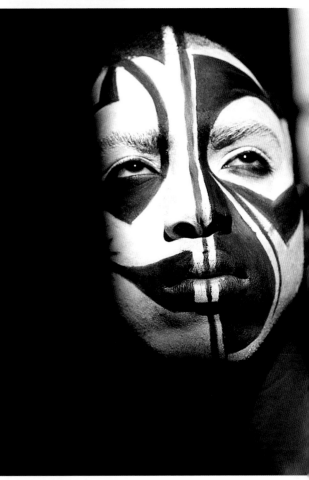

To do this Picasso/African inspired makeup on Lori (top right and above), I applied black Kryolan aquacolor to her face, leaving certain areas empty. I made paper cut-outs, then sprayed on white makeup, then the pink lips. When spraying on a color, make sure the model's eyes and mouth are closed and that his or her nostrils are covered. *Photos (top right and above) by John Chen, 1988. Hair: John Sahag.*

Copy of an original African makeup style.

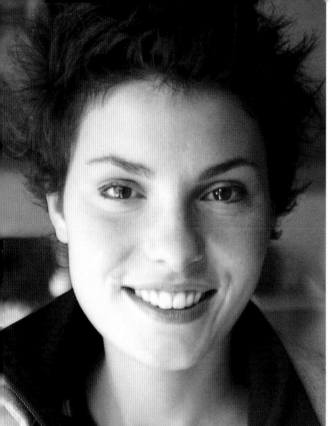

Very easy, fresh, and modern. Concealer, no base. Yellow cream shadow applied over the entire lid, with a dot of turquoise in the center of the eye. The yellow makes the turquoise more vibrant and green. *Model: Kristine.*

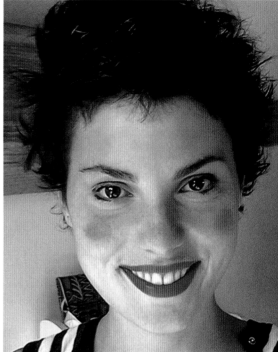

Rounds of blush.

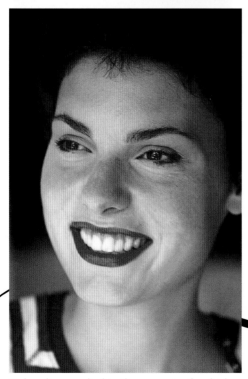

Red eyeliner applied to the eyes over the shadow.

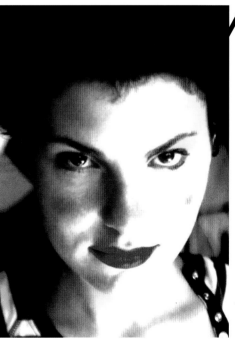

Red lipstick makes a more sophisticated look.

Brush Strokes

Dry brushes make the best strokes, and as the first strokes with a brush are the best, you need a good collection of firm brushes in various sizes. You will need to wash and dry the brush before you can use it again. It is also best to use a different brushes for each new color, unless you want to do a special stroke with two or three different colors on a brush.

When you are using Aquacolors on the face, wet the brush a little and rub it on the color or colors that you want to use. If you put more than one color on a brush, separate the bristles so that you apply one color to one section, and another to the other. That way, you have more than one color on the brush, but not on the same bristles, and when you paint with it, you'll get streaks of different color in the same stroke rather than one streak of muddy color. Freestyle makeup has much in common with painting. The effects you create are determined by the texture of the paint you use, your brushstrokes, the strength of your "lines," and your combination and placement of colors. Let yourself be inventive. As I've said, this isn't about doing makeup "right," it's about challenging yourself and trying new ways of doing something you've always done.

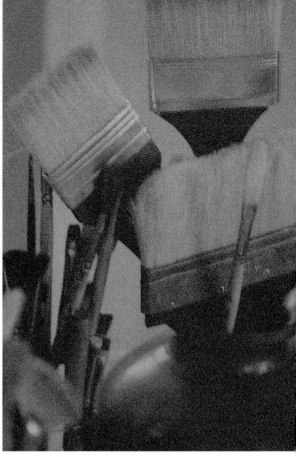

Firm paintbrushes for painting the body freestyle.

Freestyle body painting should be spontaneous and quick, so it's best to have all your materials out and ready. To save time, I use the Aquacolors by putting a portion of the product into a bowl, then pouring water a little at a time onto the product and mixing it together into a smooth paste with a paint stick or a spoon. Be careful not to make it too liquid because it will then run. This method allows me to mix colors easily like a painter would on a palette, except I am using bowls. I have lots of different bowls of color that are open enough to allow me to dip my largest brush into them. Depending on how thick your paste is, you may need to wet your brush.

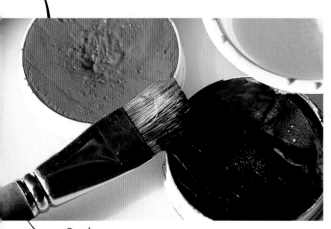

Brush.

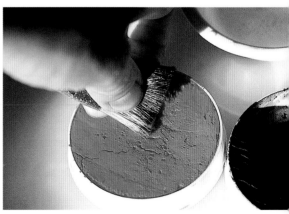

End of stroke: black-and-red line.

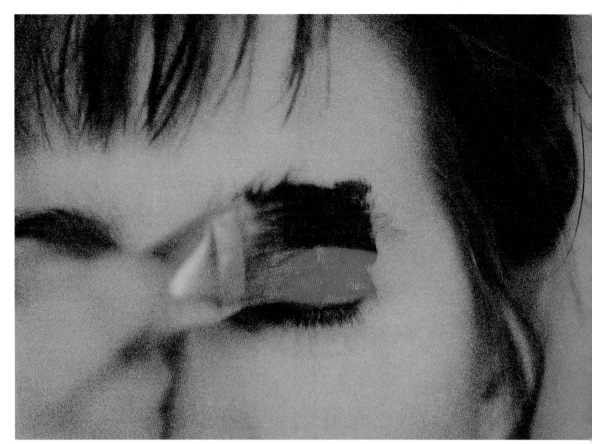

Brush with two colors.

Alice, 2002.

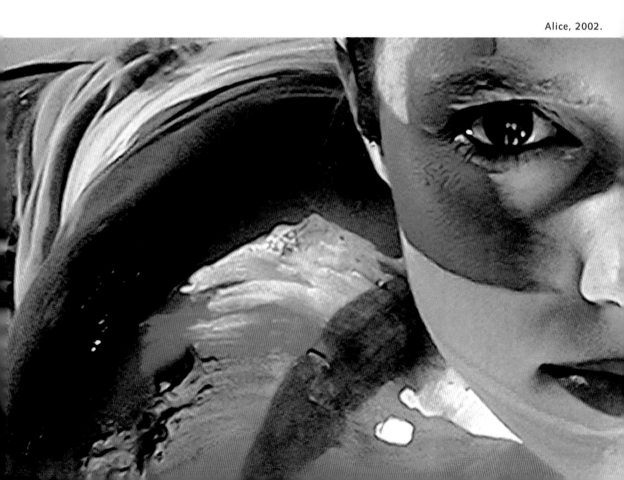

I very often work on a model while she is moving—when I see her move, her personality comes through and it inspires my choice of colors, the shape of the stroke I use, and the build-up of the colors. The body paint itself gives the suggestion of motion; the brush strokes reveal the progress of what many painters and sculptors refer to as "the hand of the artist." I like to think that if I get it right, one brush stroke will be enough for the photographer to get a great shot that captures the moment. You may want to start by painting on just one stroke when you begin doing body painting and freestyle makeup; one can be just as effective as a whole build-up of colors. Practice using the brush dry, without color, before dipping it in the pigment. Also practice doing strong swipes of color on paper; then try your first "real" stroke on your arm to see if you're getting enough color. Once you start painting, always use a different brush for each different color, or keep different colors on different sections of one brush to avoid blurring and muddying them.

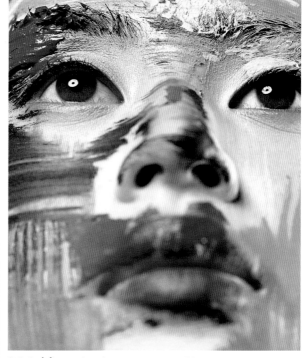

Painted face. *Photo by Bruno Gaget. Model: Minami.*

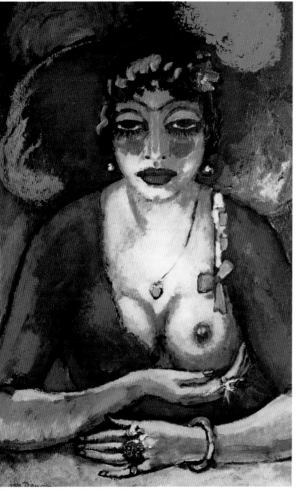

Femme Fatale, Kees Van Dongen, 1905. Oil, **31½ x 23⅝ in (80 x 60 cm)**. *© 2003 Artists Rights Society (ARS), New York/ADAGP, Paris.*

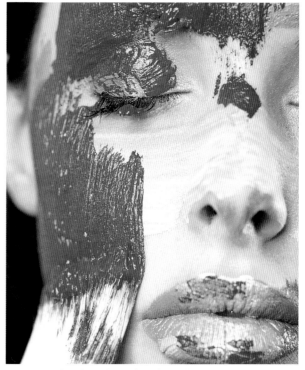

Large paintbrush stoke with red Kryolan Aquacolor. *Photo by Bruno Gaget.*

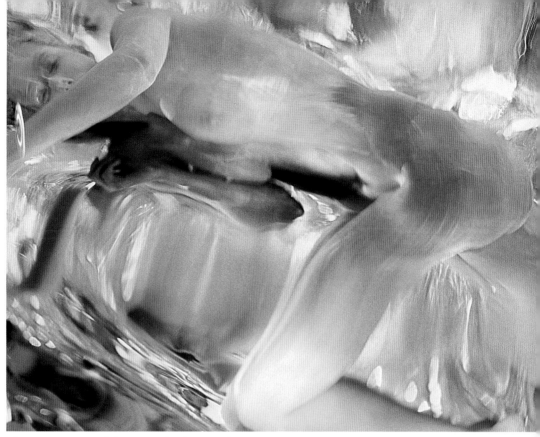

This image was used for an article about perfume. George gave me
free rein on the body painting, and his use of daylight and mirrors made the photograph
more illustrative. *"Atomic Woman"* © *photographed by George Holz for* Harper's Bazaar, *1986, all other*
rights reserved.

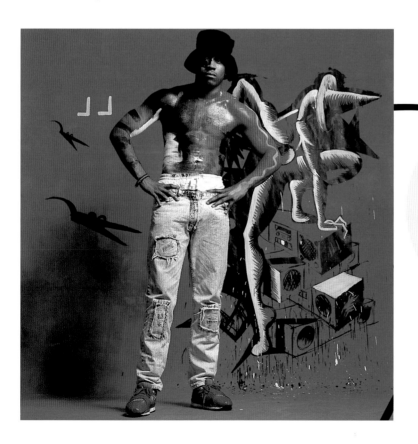

LL Cool J in freestyle body
paint for the book I did
with Seiichi Tanaka and
Marc Kostabi.
Photo by Tanaka/Mason/Kostabi.

materials

You can use almost anything to do freestyle makeup. You probably won't go out wearing jelly or flour on your face the way I have demonstrated on some of the models in these photos. You can, however, take your old eye shadow powders out of their pans and experiment with them—mix them with Vaseline or glycerin and blend them across your face. Apply pearlized shadows with a wet brush, or mix them with water and streak them across your face. Blending and smudging is best with bright creams because they do not lend themselves as well to large brush strokes. Leave creams thick, press colored eye-shadow powder into them, or blend them well to leave an almost imperceptible wash of color.

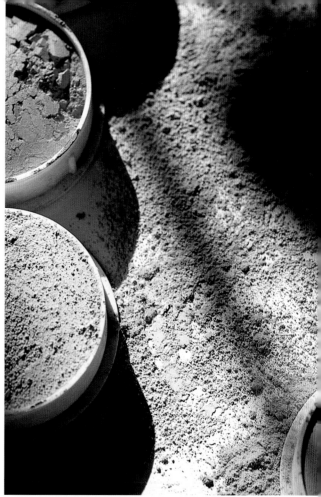

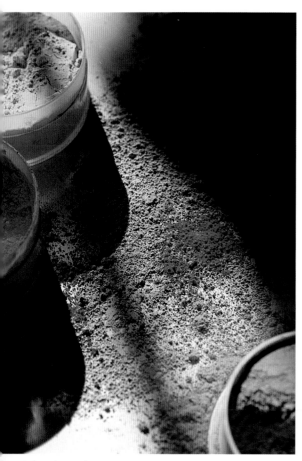

Colored powders.

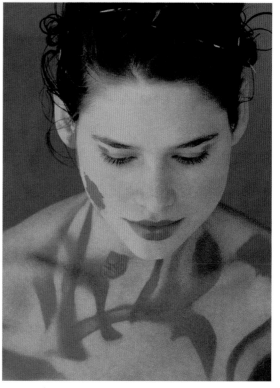

Stenciled, abstract flowers. *Photo by Roger Eaton. Hair: Gabrielle Saba for John Sahag.*

Kryolan Aquacolor is a great medium for freestyle techniques, especially body painting. The colors can be applied wet or dry with a sponge or your fingers. I like to mix them with a little water until I get a fairly stiff paste and then apply them like paint; they glide onto the skin very well with flat, firmhaired, conventional paintbrushes. Sometimes I apply one color alone, but most often I mix colors, even adding a little Day-glo at times (a kind of fluorescent, almost neon color) to brighten them up.

The paintbrushes should have fairly stiff hair so that you are able to get a strong stroke that distributes the color well, but you don't want the brush to be so hard that it scratches the skin. You should also have brushes in a variety of different sizes.

Breaking out of the mold with freestyle makeup is very liberating. You can wear it any time you feel like exercising your creative impulses or just to play. You don't have to wear it strongly and look bold and unconventional—you can also wear it delicately and transparently to add almost imperceptible touches of color to brighten your life.

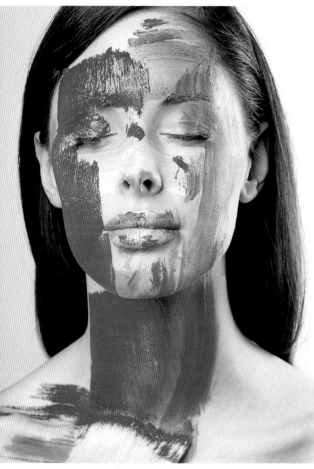

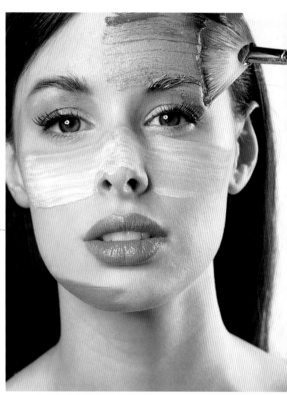

Vertical brush stroke with Japanese brush and two colors. *Photo by Bruno Gaget.*

Horizontal brush stroke with two colors.
Photo by Bruno Gaget.

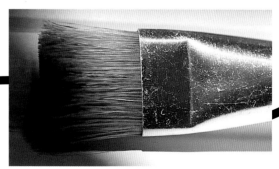

A good, firm brush for one stroke across the eyelid.

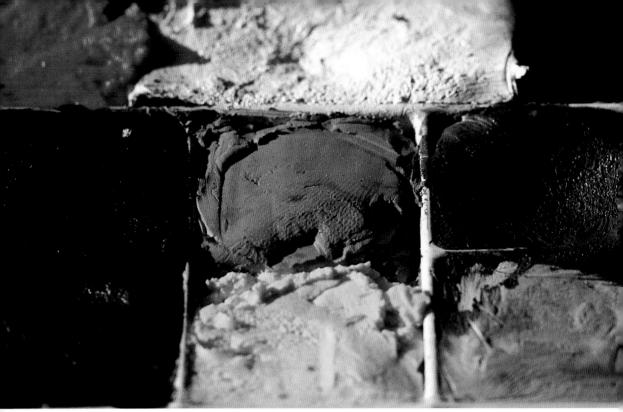

Strong pigments.

Because you cannot do large
strokes with creams, they
are better smudged or
blended on.

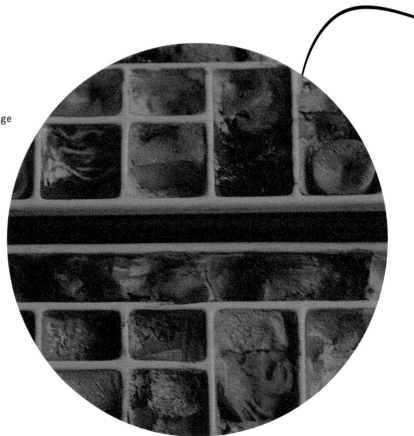

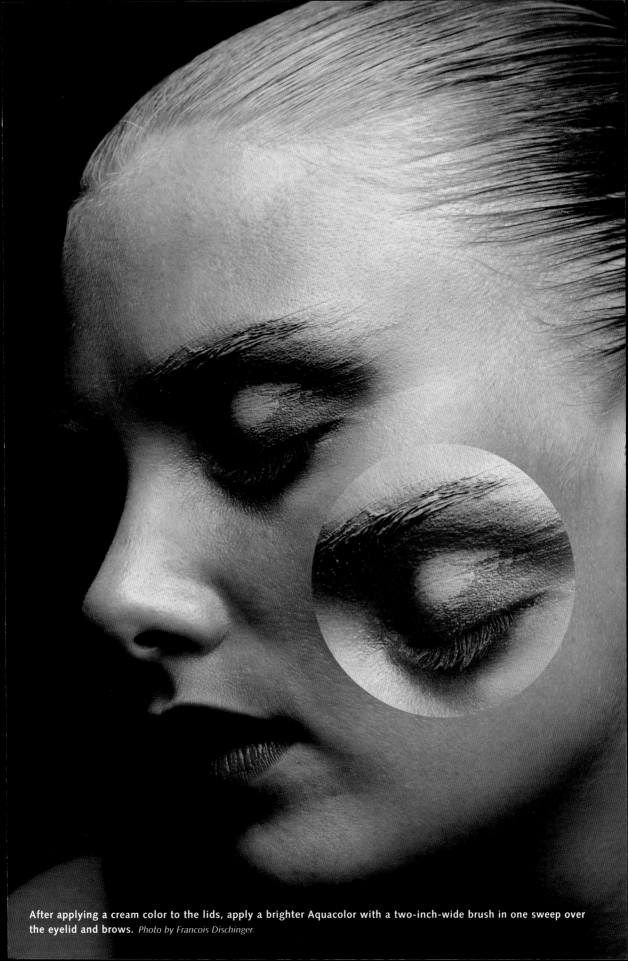

After applying a cream color to the lids, apply a brighter Aquacolor with a two-inch-wide brush in one sweep over the eyelid and brows. *Photo by Francois Dischinger.*

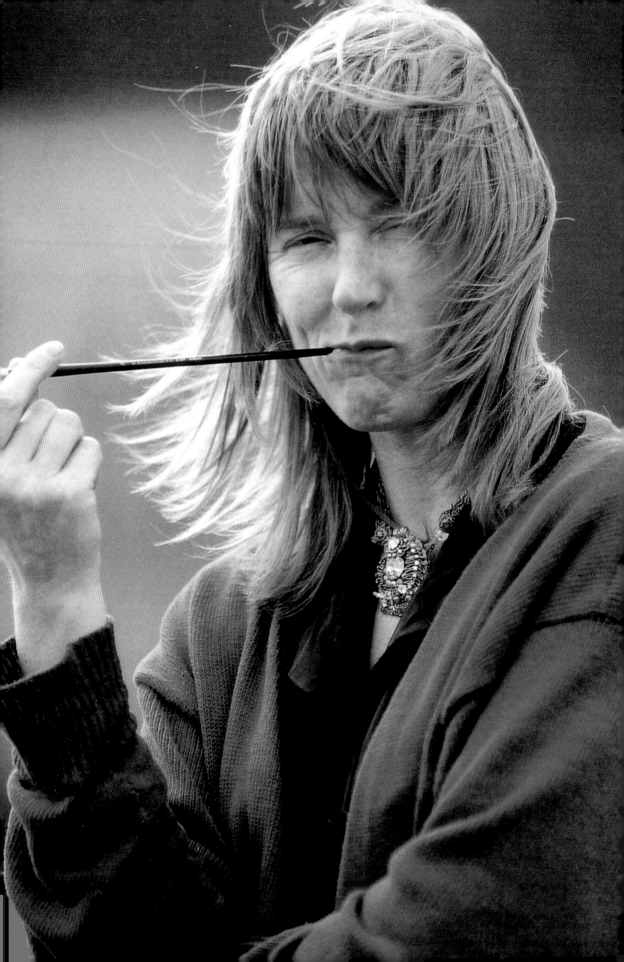

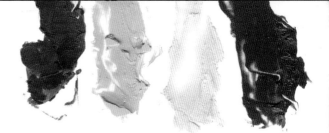

professional makeup

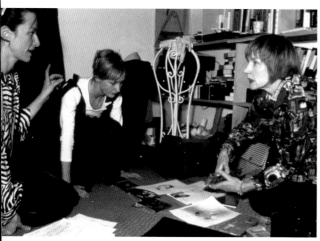

Linda Mason (right) with Cynthia Rowley (far left), preparing the makeup for her 1996 show. *Photo by David Webber.*

From the very beginning, my career as a makeup artist has always been eventful—maybe that is why I love it so much. Every situation is different, and you need to be able to act rapidly and change course if necessary to respond to things like models not showing up for jobs, jobs that are booked at the last minute, or accidentally being booked for two jobs at once.

One example of the unpredictable nature of this line of work took place when I was working with the photographer Claus Wickrath on a magazine spread. A shoot for an Italian magazine was supposed to be going on in the studio next door, but they had lost their model and photographer. The magazine's editor was stuck there with the clothes, thinking she had wasted a great deal of time and money. Susan, the very ambitious model Claus and I had hired, chatted with the magazine editor and came back and begged Claus and me to do that shoot with her after we had finished our own. Well, we finished our job at 7 P.M. and then worked all night on the other shoot—I left at 9 A.M. the next morning and had to go straight to my next booking for that day. Susan, the model, was a real pro; even though she was so tired she kept falling asleep, she wouldn't give up until the work was finished. *Neither can you:* that's my purpose for sharing this story. If you really want to be a makeup artist, you should be aware that there are many kinds of assignments that require you to work hard in all kinds of circumstances at unpredictable hours. However, there are also plenty of other kinds of work in the field that allow you to have more control over your environment. Knowing what to expect and how to prepare yourself for the various scenarios in which you may work will allow you to make the most of this adventure.

Linda Mason on location in the Canary Islands with Hans Feurer for Italian *Vogue*. *Photo by Hans Feurer.*

optimum work conditions

Comfortable conditions and good lighting are essential in any makeup room, whether it's your personal or work space. You should be comfortable and relaxed, so when you're working on your own makeup, it's better to sit than to stand. Bending towards the mirror or down towards the counter or dresser where you keep all your makeup creates strain, which interferes with the efficient progression of your work. Good positioning and good posture are important; you will just enjoy doing makeup more if you're comfortable. When you have to stand to work on a client or model, wear flat shoes. Having a chair whose height you can adjust is ideal for working on clients. All this may sound like common sense, but it will probably take you a while to arrange your work space for optimum comfort and function.

If you're working at a shoot or a fashion show, don't be afraid to ask for a better chair if the one you have been given is not right. The model must be comfortable, too; otherwise she will be squirming around, making your job difficult. If you are right-handed, as I am, set up all your materials to your right; if you're left-handed, obviously, set them up on your left.

Having the model sit in front of a mirror enables you to see your work reflected at you, but this method also has the disadvantage of also allowing the model to see what you are

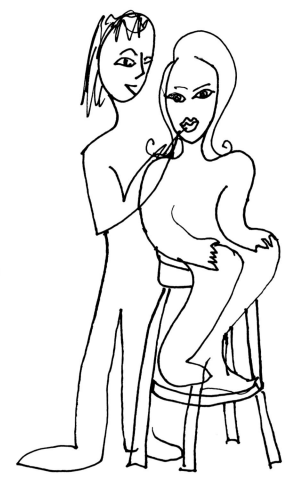

doing. If you are just "getting to know" her face, you will go through some trial and error, and having her watch you could break your concentration. If she sees you "trying" a few things, she might start to feel insecure and uneasy. I started out only being able to work with the model facing a mirror, and I worked for many years this way, often stepping back behind the model and looking straight into the mirror at her to check my work. I now prefer to have my model facing good light, preferably daylight. If you have your model facing a mirror, the "temperature" of the light (a term photographers use to refer to the intensity and degree of light) should be as near as possible to a clear-skied, daytime lighting; makeup under these conditions will appear as well under daylight as artificial light. Frontal lighting is best. If your model is facing a mirror, the lights should extend along the top and down the sides of the mirror. Beware of overhead lighting: if it is positioned *directly* overhead, it will create shadows on the face, and you'll either have to move your model or turn the lights off.

As soon as I arrive in the studio, I immediately look for a place to set up in the flattest daylight possible; however, you don't want bright sunlight shining directly onto the position. If you can't avoid that, use a transparent white curtain to cut down the light, otherwise you, the model, and your products will melt.

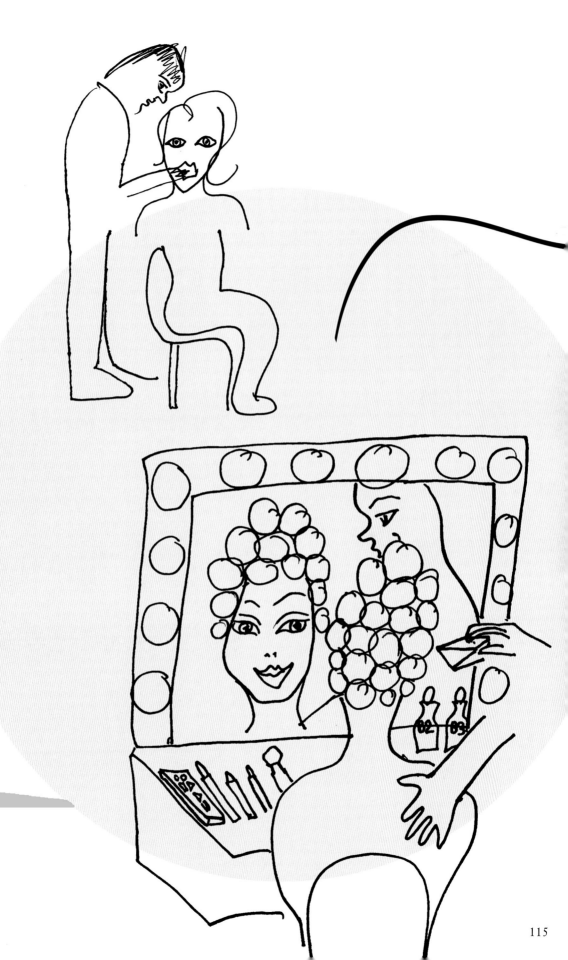

115

magazine work

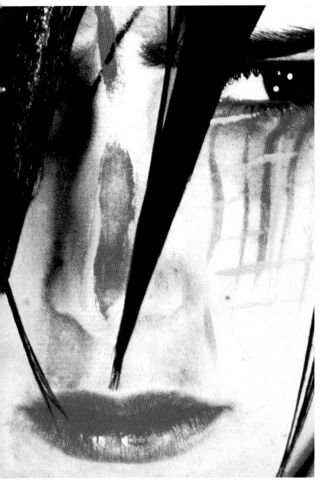

A fun fashion editorial. *Photo by Jean Jacques Castres.*

There are several kinds of editorial work, which involves a photo shoot that appears in a magazine. A **"fashion editorial"** is about clothing—the models' faces are not usually photographed up-close; a **"beauty editorial"** is about a particular beauty theme, such as hair, skin care, or makeup, and it focuses on the models' faces.

Many magazines use photographs to illustrate stories and articles that have nothing to do with fashion or beauty. The purpose of these photos is to impart atmosphere rather than to illustrate information about a product or the latest "look," so a makeup artist gets more creative freedom for such shoots. You will probably get your first chance to do magazine work for an illustration editorial because there are fewer constraints; thus, the editor is under less pressure and more willing to take a risk.

The pay for editorial work varies, but as a rule, it is significantly less than that for advertising or catalogue shoots. However, you must do editorial work if you want to get the better-paying jobs. You will be able not only to build a better portfolio to show to advertising agencies but also to get immense exposure to the people in the industry. You will be out and about meeting more and more great models, hairstylists, and stylists, and they will in turn be able to recommend *you* when *they* are booked on better-paying jobs.

When I first started doing makeup for magazines, there were no agents for makeup and hair, so I spent a lot of my time calling beauty editors and art directors to get editorial work. This entailed trying to arrange meetings with them so they could see my portfolio, which, although it wasn't very big at the time, was still presentable. I did have a lot of tests and photos from a couple of jobs I had done thanks to different contacts. Besides calling the editors, I also called photographers whose work I admired and let them know I was available to do makeup "testing" and work.

Today an aspiring makeup artist in the fashion/beauty industry *must* have an agent. With an agent, you come across as professional and experienced; without one, you'd better have an enormous pool of personal contacts and references at your disposal. A magazine will automatically ask you who your agent is; a good one has relationships with editors and other people in the business and helps introduce you to them and get you work. To find an agent, check the magazines to see which makeup artists' work you admire—the name of the agent is often printed next to the artist's. To see which agencies represent photographers you like, check out the photographer on the Internet and ask them which makeup agencies they would recommend. There is also a publication called *The Black Book* that lists agents.

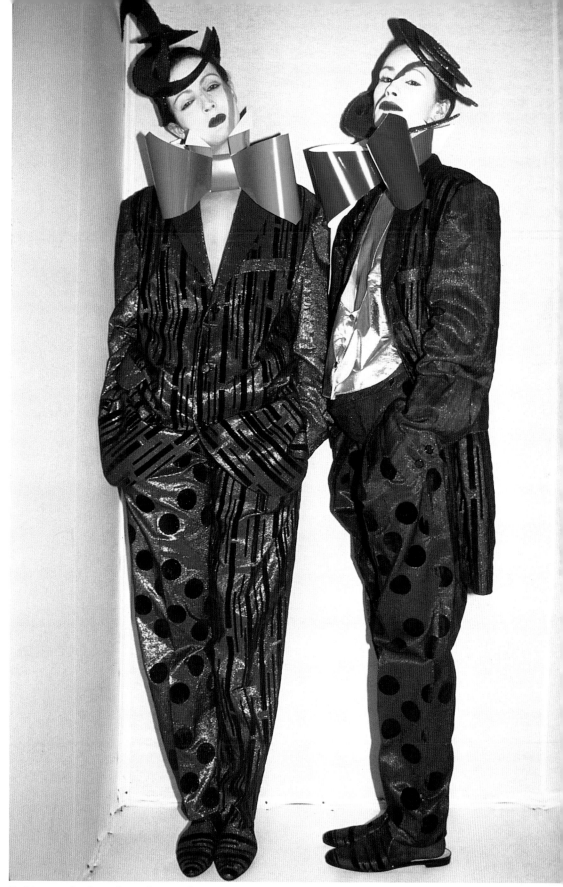

Fashion article about the makeup and clothing at the 1982 France Andrevie show. *Photo by Roxanne Lowit, 1982.*

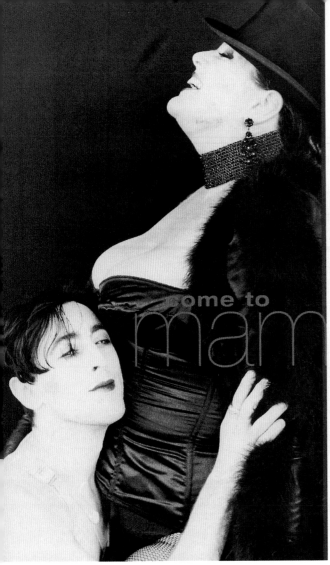

ome to

mama.

"I met Camryn on the set of *Romy and Michele's High School Reunion*," says *Cabaret* star Alan Cumming. "We were having lunch when I told her she had spinach between her teeth. We immediately became friends. Now I call her the oracle of New York because she knows everyone here. And because I hang out with her, so do I."

Camryn Manheim and Alan Cumming for MODE.
Photo by Gerhard Yurkovic, 1998.

Worth & Worth top hat. Miguel Ases at Fragments long bead earrings and bead choker. La Crasia leather gloves. Frederick's of Hollywood satin corset. Fernando Sanchez silk dressing gown.

Having an agent does not mean you shouldn't also cultivate contacts with photographers, editors, and art directors on your own. Every contact you can establish in the business is important. Find out what your agent's plan of action is and whether there's something you can do to help.

It's difficult to say who has the most influence on whether or not you get jobs. In some cases, the photographer has the most say, especially if he or she has a strong style and is well respected. For a beauty article, a magazine's beauty editor will definitely have the last word, but he or she will either book a photographer who works with a team (hair stylists and makeup artists) that she knows, or choose a team with the photographer.

You can often be more creative when working with fashion editors than with beauty editors. Beauty articles are also the most difficult to do because they involve more than just makeup application—they must also convey certain information to the reader. As a makeup artist, you have to be able to contribute to the article as a whole; you're not just making the models look pretty. Therefore, an editor needs to know that you will be able to satisfy all her needs. It may even be that you contribute to the idea of the beauty story. Or, when you do fashion shoots for certain magazines, the pictures may end up being used for beauty stories or even for the cover.

Discovering Beauty

Try not to be judgmental about beauty. To this day, I am still astounded by the way some women, who seem plain at first or even almost ugly when you study them in detail become more and more beautiful the more you "discover" what brings those features to life and the mysterious qualities that can be incredible in front of the camera.

The perfect model, photogenic from any angle and perfectly at ease and comfortable with herself, is extremely rare. The majority of models are beautiful, but not from any angle, and they may not have such secure personalities. As one of the first people to work with the models, it is the makeup artist's job to help put them at ease. Watch for signs of facial tension of which you can try to make the model aware and try to find ways to help her relax.

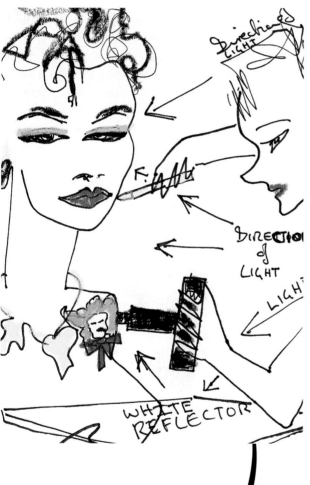

Just as you search a little to find the right makeup, the photographer will often need time to figure out the best lighting for the model. Certain photographers have a particular lighting they feel comfortable using in most situations. If you see that the model doesn't look too good in that light, you have to adjust the makeup to suit it. I often like to work on the set where I can see the model in the light, rather than doing it beforehand. I recommend this if you are trying to do something a little unusual or creative. Models can become intimidated by this type of makeup and lose their sense of freedom and spontaneity, which is important for a successful shoot.

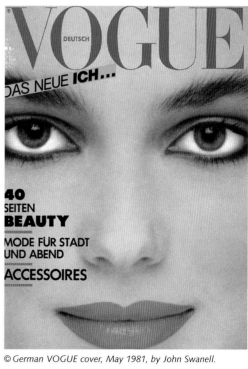

© German VOGUE cover, May 1981, by John Swanell.

119

working on location

Some people thrive on the unpredictable: 4 A.M. calls, early morning rides through dark forests or jungles, and freshly caught fish barbecued on the beach. Others hate to get up early and are cranky when they can't find their usual coffee and a bagel. Working on location puts you in lots of unpredictable situations. If you're one of the latter, you'll have a rough adjustment if you pursue such assignments. Fortunately I am one of the former and have enjoyed many interesting adventures throughout my career.

There are four different types of location shoots: advertising, catalogue, editorial, and commercial or music video. Each requires a different approach.

- When doing a product **advertising shoot**, you are often making up only one person over a period of a few days with the same makeup. Once you've decided upon the best makeup for the project, you must often make up that person the same way every day. You do the makeup once in the morning and once in the afternoon, with lots of touch-ups in between. Constant touch-ups are necessary because of the difficulties imposed by the elements (you're working outdoors) and the physical exertion often required of the model in an outdoor setting, such as running, playing in the waves, and so on.

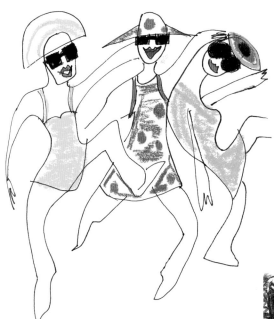

When I did my first photo shoots for ELLE magazine in 1975, I was quite ignorant about who the different photographers were and what was expected of me, and I was lucky they asked me back. I did very strong makeup on the models in beautiful shades of orange and pink; however, they were wearing little summer dresses. Had I checked out the photographer (Toscani's) work first, I would have seen that his laughing, smiling, jumping girls needed much more subtle makeup. A true professional, he rescued both the photos and me by putting sunglasses on the girls in every picture.

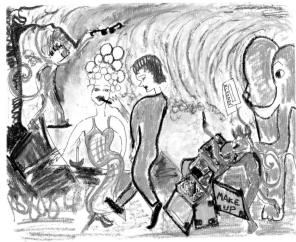

I drew this when I was working on location in Zambia, a place I loved, especially for the people, the animals, and the beautiful Victoria Falls. Before leaving Paris, the photographer for the shoot purchased some new sunglasses, and he aggravated all of us by never taking them off. On the evening of the second day of the photo shoot, everyone sat down by the river watching the hippopotami, and a monkey swung down from a tree, swiped the sunglasses off the photographer's face, and threw them in the river.

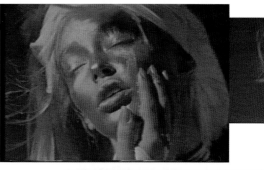

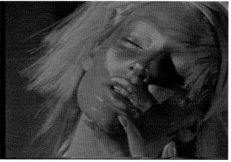

- **Catalogue (also know as fashion advertising) shoots** are usually more intense than those for product advertising. Often there are more than three models, sometimes as many as five or six, for whom you must decide upon and apply a makeup. After every picture, there will be a location change. The makeup is often altered to accommodate that, so you must be fast and organized.

- Location shoots for **magazine editorials** are similar to fashion advertising shoots in that there are usually three models and there is a lot to do. However, they differ in that the atmosphere is a bit looser and they permit more creative freedom. Usually, all the beauty articles and maybe a couple of fashion shoots for one month's issue offor are done over the course of three days to a week, sometimes more, sometimes less, so it's early to rise and late to bed. It's often like a week-long, exhausting party full of surprises.

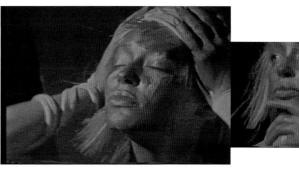

Stills taken from a music video by director Ken Ross and art director Paula Grief.

- **Commercials and music videos** are also often shot on location. These productions usually involve many more people, but you may be booked to make up just one of the featured celebrities or models, and another makeup artist may be booked for the others. If you have more than one person to look after, if possible, bring one or more assistants with you. Someone must always be present on the set, and you may need help restocking or with various other tasks. On music videos, you should be prepared to work all night, with long periods of waiting around followed by intense activity, but this kind of work can be lots of fun. You can be very creative, and although you still have to be careful and consistent, continuity (doing the same makeup) is usually not as important as it is in commercials.

When you arrive on location, it's best to meet with the photographer and stylist or editor prior to shooting to discuss the direction in which they'd like to go. This means you get a chance to see the models and the clothing. Occasionally you will have a photographer who wants you to do a test the day before. I have been on a couple trips when, unfortunately, the test days were the only ones for which we had good weather. Often you can spend three days shooting, only to have to reshoot everything the fourth day because someone found a more inspiring location or because the weather improved.

Working on Location in the City

Going on location doesn't necessarily mean going to exotic places—most often, it will mean working from a van in the town in which you work. When I first started out as a makeup artist, I must admit I felt more comfortable in the studio because of its controlled environment. Once I became more confident with my makeup, I began to prefer working on location.

If you have more than one girl to do, you should finish the first girl, then try to get all the other models partially done before the photographer leaves the van to start shooting the first model, when you must go with him. Once you have checked the first girl on the set, ask the photographer if you can run back to the van to finish the next girl. This is only possible if you're working on a fashion shoot; on a beauty shoot, you have to stay with the photographer because you have to keep a very close eye on the model's face. A multitude of things could very easily happen: a simple gust of wind could blow dust on the model's face; her hair could blow onto her lips, smudge the makeup, and ruin the picture; if she's in the wind or sun, her eyes could become red and teary and ruin the eye makeup, or it could fade or run.

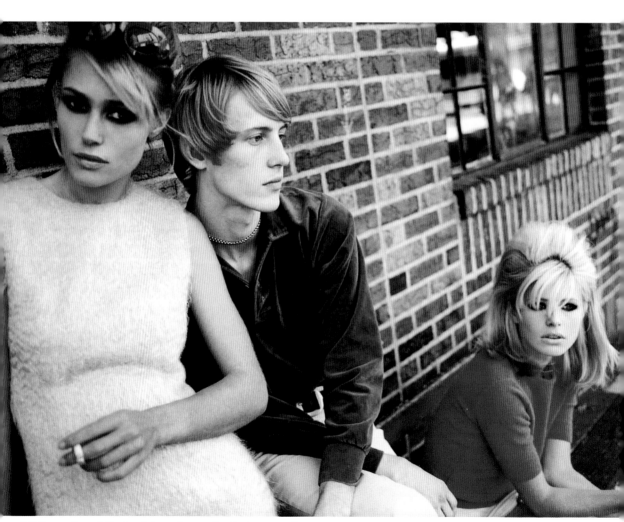

A '90s version of the Bardot smoky eye for *Amica* magazine. *Photos by Alessandro D'Andrea, 1995. Stylist: Cinzia Brandi.*

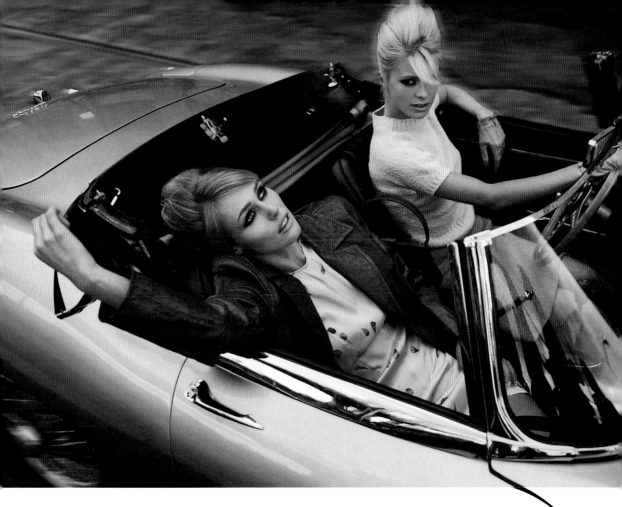

Typically, when you work on location outside in the city, you shoot winter clothes in summer and summer clothes in winter because of the three months it takes to produce the magazine. In summer, those winter clothes can make the models perspire; in winter, the exposure to the cold gives the models red noses and hands. To counteract perspiration, you should always blot the model's face with tissue paper first, *before* reapplying powder, to avoid build-up. After blotting, you may find you don't need to reapply powder. Each model is different, and usually, those who drink a lot of water need the most attention because they perspire more. The red nose is a more difficult problem; the only solution is to apply a base that has heavier-than-normal coverage.

If the model is not able to wear gloves, you may need to make up her hands and have her shake them in the air to get the circulation going before the photographer starts shooting. Some people just have hands that are naturally redder than other people's, and though a heavy base on the hands isn't terribly attractive, in some cases it's necessary. Discuss this with the photographer because he or she knows how this will look on film and will make a note of it when taking the shot.

Always be organized: the van might have to change locations, and you must be prepared to close up your material quickly.

Working on Location in Hot Climates

When I'm working outside in hot weather, whether in an exotic location or just the nearby countryside, I set up my kit not too far from where the photographer is shooting, preferably under a tree or otherwise away from the direct sunlight, and let myself enjoy the benefits of all the space, light, and fresh air.

Unfortunately, the models will often need to be ready for the camera by daybreak (which is the hour with the best light, according to many photographers). Depending on how remote and exotic your location is, this may mean working under some unusual conditions, such as having to do makeup by candlelight, as I had to do once on location in Africa. If at all possible, find time the day before the shoot to do test makeup or at least to check the models' skin and features so you know what you will be dealing with. Working outside on location means working in an *uncontrolled environment*. Take advantage of the few things you *can* control and then just take the rest as it comes.

Matching the Makeup to the Setting

Get as much information about the shoot ahead of time as possible—it will save you a lot of trouble later on. Many shoots will take place on the beach, and the models will be in the water; you'll need to bring waterproof mascara as well as waterproof bases and blushes. The models will usually be in shallow water very close to the photographer and you, and you will have to touch up their makeup whenever it shows signs of dissolving. Water can make the skin look great, but it does not hide its imperfections. Unless your model has flawless skin, you need to disguise uneven areas and dark undereye circles with a waterproof foundation or concealer. Custom-mix the concealer so that it matches the model's skin tone or is a shade lighter. It's best to do so in natural rather than artificial light because that's the best way to really test the match and, after all, you will be shooting outside in natural light. You don't want the makeup to be darker or pinker than the model's natural skin tone. If you ever need to make a correction on the base in the daylight, remove the unwanted patch with a Q-tip dipped in cleanser, wipe the spot with toner or water, then reapply the concealer/base mix in the same light. Many models tan their bodies but not their faces; you'll need to use a warmer shade of base to bring the face up to match the body. If the shoot is in a warm climate, the model is usually asked to actually get a tan before a shoot by either using a tanning bed or sunbathing. In this situation, your job will be to enhance the tan and make it look even. If a model has fair skin, you can deepen the color with a tinted moisturizer or a colored sunscreen like the orange gelee made by Bain de Soleil. (This product gives skin a wonderful glow.) Always apply tinted moisturizer and sunscreen before you apply any concealer or base. You won't know how long the model will have to be out in the sun, and although most models just want to tan as quickly as possible, few realize how quickly a tan can go red in the blazing sun during a shoot. A slight glow is attractive in a photo, but a sunburn is not. (Not to mention the fact that burning damages the skin in many ways.)

Keep your eye on the models between photos as well. You do not want them getting too much sun exposure or tan lines, which are difficult to cover.

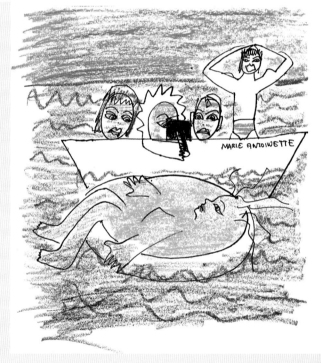

MARIE ANTOIWETTE

124

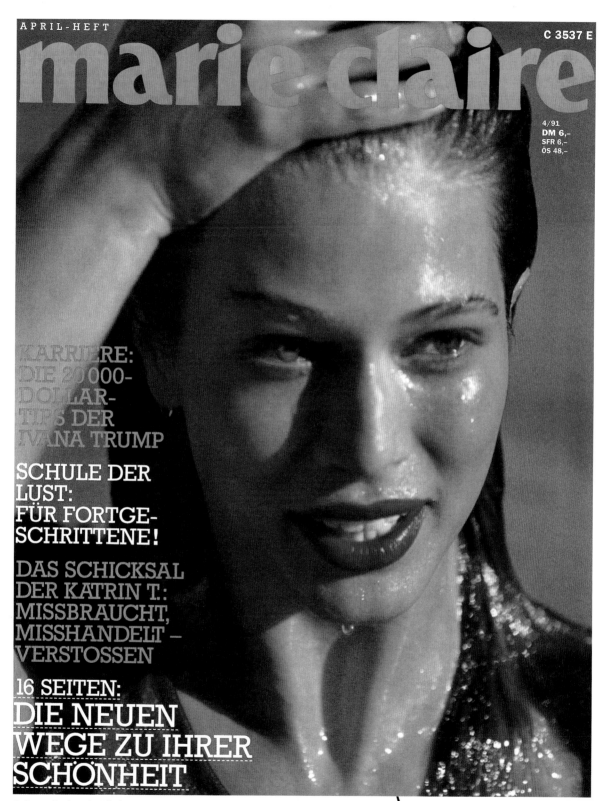

APRIL-HEFT

C 3537 E

marie claire

4/91
DM 6,–
SFR 6,–
ÖS 48,–

KARRIERE:
DIE 20000-
DOLLAR-
TIPS DER
IVANA TRUMP

SCHULE DER
LUST:
FÜR FORTGE-
SCHRITTENE!

DAS SCHICKSAL
DER KATRIN T.:
MISSBRAUCHT,
MISSHANDELT –
VERSTOSSEN

16 SEITEN:
DIE NEUEN
WEGE ZU IHRER
SCHÖNHEIT

Actress Amber Smith for German *Marie Claire*. This is an example of an outdoor, on-location shot in which the model needed to look tanned. I applied suntan lotion to her skin and a little concealer under her eyes. I used a deep lip shade applied sparingly to emphasize her great lips.
Photo by William Garrett, 1992.

What to Bring to Work in Any Weather

Location shootings in exotic climates do not always take place in bright sunlight—you may find yourself in torrential rains, freezing snow, or a even an earthquake—but the shoot must always go on. The photographer cannot leave the shoot until he has all the photos he needs, so be prepared to work in some challenging conditions and see some odd things.

A makeup box that's comfortable to sit on when it's closed is a lifesaver when you're traveling. I stow odds and ends that don't go in the case in washable plastic makeup bags, but when I travel, I pack whatever does go in the makeup case in a plastic bag as well in case of spills. When I started, I would take a fairly large makeup case, but I have learned to take a much smaller one to accommodate all the climbing and walking I may have to do. I also have a large, waterproof shoulder bag (a backpack works well, too) that is great to just throw everything into when I need to move on speedily. Other makeup artists swear by the plastic roll-up cosmetic bags. I find them easy to carry, but inconvenient to work with; I like to just dive into my open box and take out what I need. The bags are more difficult to get into, you have to fish around for what you need, and, being plastic, they can get awfully hot in the sun.

When traveling by plane, take your box with you as a carry-on item. *Don't check it as baggage.* You can always borrow or buy clothes if your suitcase goes astray, but you will not have the time to find and stock a new makeup case if yours is lost.

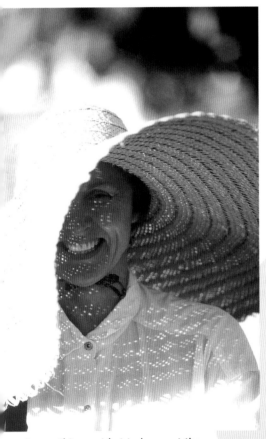

I wore this great hat to keep out the sun when I was on location in the Canary Islands for Italian *Vogue.*

Photos (both pages) by Hans Feurer.
Stylist: Caroline Baker.

Location Checklist

Hot Climate	Cold Climate
Sun hat	Warm hat
Self-tanning lotion	Heavy moisturizer
Cotton swabs	Cotton swabs
Sponges	Sponges
Bathing suit	Long johns and thermals
Insect repellant	Gloves
Sunglasses	Blanket
Tissues	Heavy bases
Powder puffs	Sketches and/or Polaroids of everything necessary, boxes, bags, etc.
Sun block in SPF 30 and 15	
Waterproof tan cream	
Cleanser	
Cotton balls	
Towel	

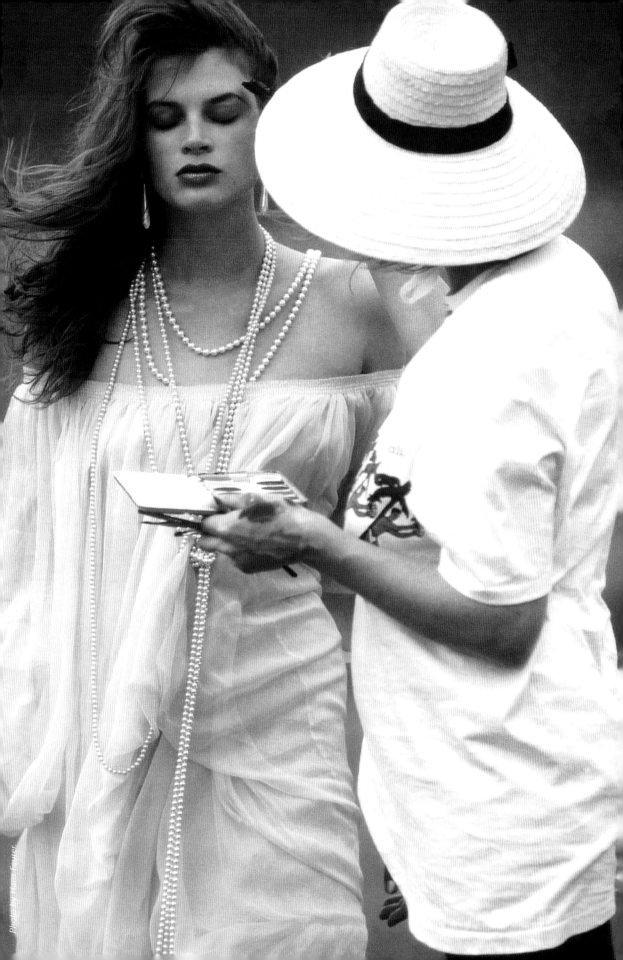

fashion shows

There are lots of opportunities for new makeup artists to get work doing runway shows. They can either try to make connections with young designers themselves or work as assistants for more experienced artists.

Fashion shows are incredibly inspiring and full of a great energy. You get to work with a cast of very talented people in a team dynamic. Runway shows are much bigger productions than photo shoots. The pace of the environment is much faster and often, everyone is *frantic*. If you're working with a young designer who is just starting out, you may be paid a minimal sum—sometimes you'll be paid with merchandise. That is fine, and to be expected, but not if the designer has managed to find the money to pay the models a fortune. You may choose to find a sponsor who will pay to have your name credited in association with theirs. When I did my first show in Paris with the designer Angelo Tarlazzi, I worked with one of the top runway models of the period, Anna Pavlotti. She spoke to all the designers about me, and soon I was working with all the designers for whom she was doing shows. At that time I was working for Helena Rubinstein, so I didn't need to find a sponsor.

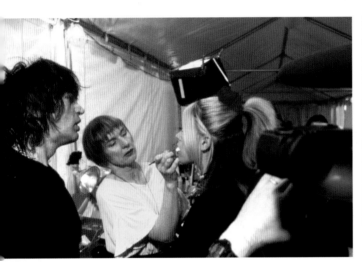

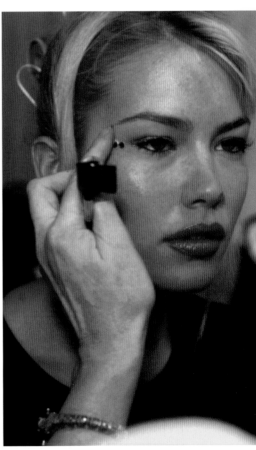

Back stage at the Cynthia Rowley show with hairstylist John Sahag. I wanted the models to look like they had done their makeup themselves, so I put together a kit for each girl the way I did when I started in the '70s.
Photos by David Webber.

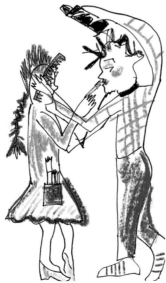

Makeup artist and hairstylist.

Finishing off the model's violet eye makeup with jewels before she goes on stage.

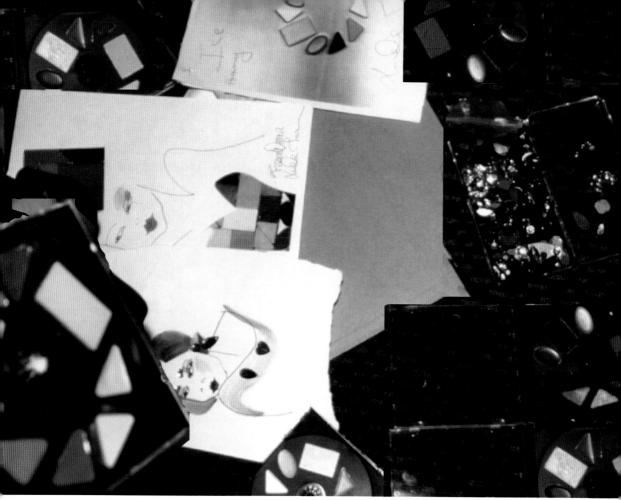

Proposals for color palettes, sketches, and materials for the Cynthia Rowley show.

You will probably have at least one meeting, if not more, with the fashion designer before their show to do a test makeup. At your first meeting, you will look at the actual clothes or see sketches of them. The designer might have an idea for a "face" he or she thinks would work with the clothes. If you have an idea comes to you immediately, see if you can test it on someone who works in the designer's studio. If you can't, work on some sketches of your ideas, or try them on your friends. Come back and present the ideas through a demonstration or your sketches. Sometimes it is quite difficult to get a feeling for a designer's style; even the successful ones occasionally have seasons when it's difficult to pinpoint the essence of the clothes. Once season it only took me a few minutes to decide on the makeup for the late French designer France Andrevie's collection, her direction was so strong. But the following collection was a disaster, and my makeup was, too.

When doing runway work, listen to the designer, but it should be clear that *you* are the makeup artist. Remember, you are the expert (or should be), so if you are not in agreement with the designer about the makeup, explain what you want to do and why it would be better for their designs. If they have an idea that's great but rather complicated and they don't have a budget for assistants, figure out a way of simplifying things. Successful designers who have been working for some time usually have a "signature" style, but you can still be creative within its framework. Makeup for fashion shows can be very avant-garde and unusual. If the models put the clothes on fairly soon after the makeup is applied, they can see and get a feeling for the total look they're showcasing. They will be more confident, and your work will be a lot easier. You should always *recheck* the models, especially the first girl you've done; in all that extra time she spends waiting, she sometimes accidentally messes up her makeup.

Another very important piece of advice for working fashion shows is to stay in the wings during the show (unless the designer tells you otherwise) and to be very attentive. Anything could happen. You may need to add makeup or add or remove body paint for an upcoming outfit. You may have to improvise on the look you've chosen as the show progresses. Even if you don't need to do any of these things, the models often need their faces blotted or powdered and their lips touched up because of the heat. It is important that you are present, but keep out of the way and don't make the models late for their next calls. Let them change their clothes first, then touch them up as they line up to go on stage.

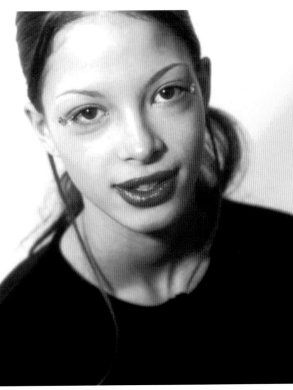

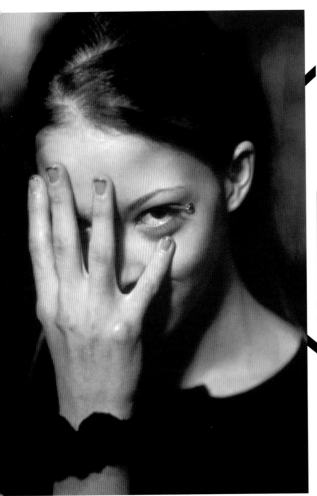

Relaxed moments back stage at the Cynthia Rowley show.
Photos by David Webber.

advertising and other Commercial Work

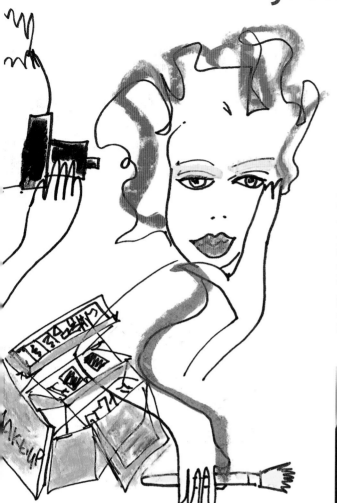

There are two different kinds of commercial work: fashion advertising and product advertising. Doing the makeup for product advertisements, particularly for cosmetics companies, is an interesting source of work. Cosmetics companies often have huge advertising budgets. They hire outside agencies to produce sophisticated ads that show off their products in the best possible light, often relying on top models, photographers, hairstylists, and *of course*, makeup artists to do that. These ads are usually placed in major, national magazines. Cosmetic companies also often do press photographs, which are separate from their main advertising photographs. These photos are only sent to the industry press to announce the company's new cosmetic products and colors. A company's principal advertising campaign, however, is usually handled by an agency.

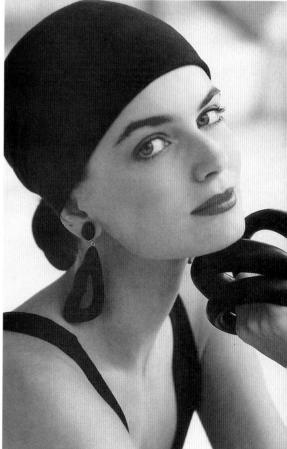

I rarely used base on Paulina Poriskova because she had such great skin.
Photo by Arthur Elgort for Anne Klein, 1985.

You could also do an advertising shoot for a brand of cigarettes or alcohol. Doing ads for cosmetics and these other products is the most lucrative, but campaigns for everything from floor polish to stereos often require makeup artists. When you're doing the makeup for any product advertisement, understand its basic concept. Get a sense of the kind of character the model or actor is portraying in the ad (a mother, a businessman, an "average Joe") and tailor the makeup to reflect that character. If you're doing an ad campaign for a bank, you want the models to look like everyday, real people, so, unless the client specifically requests a different look, keep the makeup simple. If you're doing a product ad for a cosmetics company, you will have discussions with the advertising agency's art director and talk with the photographer to find out how your work can convey the concept of the ad.

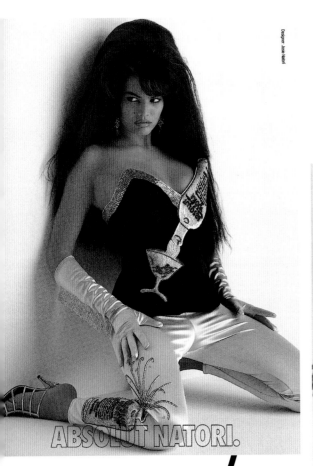

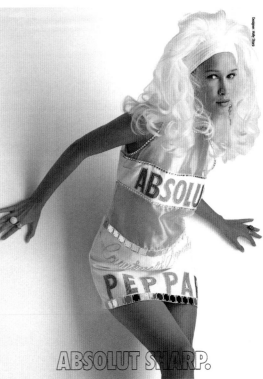

This ad campaign for Absolut Vodka featured fashions of different designers with different models.
Photo shoot with Walter Chin for Absolut Vodka, 1992.

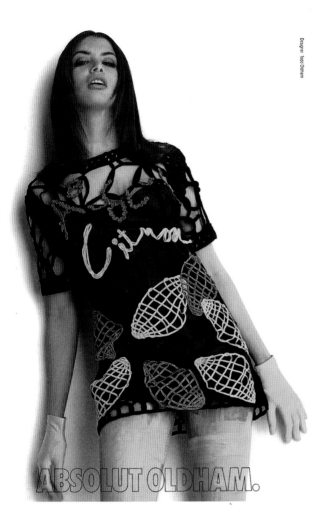

ABSOLUT OLDHAM.

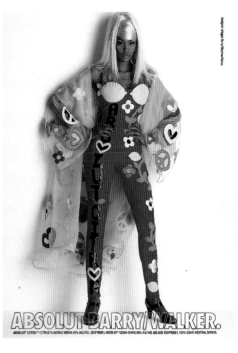

ABSOLUT BARRY/WALKER.

ABSOLUT® CITRON™—CITRUS FLAVORED VODKA 40% ALC/VOL. (80 PROOF). ABSOLUT® VODKA 40 AND 50% ALC/VOL. (80 AND 100 PROOF). 100% GRAIN NEUTRAL SPIRITS.

In Paris I worked with an incredible commercial director, Lester Bookbinder. I loved working with him, but he always seemed to have problems with hairstylists, so when he asked me to recommend someone, it was with great reticence that I did so. The hairstylist Yannick was great, but at that time I did not know he had no experience with film. It was a hair commercial, and we were to shoot one girl on a seat turning slowly around for two days, so continuation was very important. Towards the end of the second day, as we looked at the rushes from the previous day, we saw that Yannick had changed the hair. Lester asked him why he had done this. Yannick replied that he preferred it that way. Lester asked him three times if he was sure that was how he preferred it, and three times he answered "Yes." So Lester then announced that we were going to reshoot everything. We worked throughout the night reshooting everything we had done the two previous days.

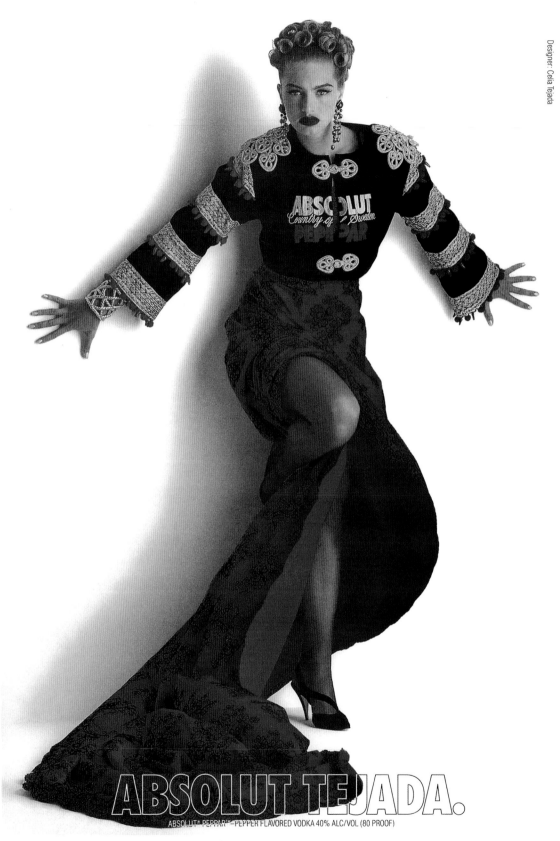

Designer: Celia Tejada

ABSOLUT TEJADA.

ABSOLUT® PEPPAR® PEPPER FLAVORED VODKA 40% ALC/VOL (80 PROOF)

Photos (both pages) by Walter Chin for same campaign for Absolut Vodka, 1992.

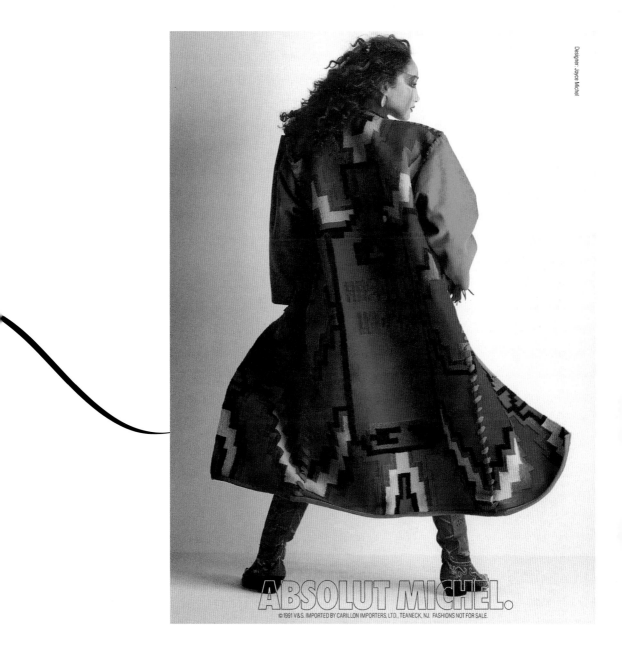

ABSOLUT MICHEL.

© 1991 V&S. IMPORTED BY CARILLON IMPORTERS, LTD., TEANECK, NJ. FASHIONS NOT FOR SALE.

When working on a television commercial, continuity is important. You do one makeup, and then keep it clean and fresh and basically the same on the model for the rest of the filming day. Sometimes you need to do the same makeup and keep it consistent for a few days in a row (unless the commercial shows different times of day and different situations, in which case other makeup may be appropriate). Maintaining continuity in the makeup is not as easy as it sounds—still photos can be retouched if you need to fix something but that is much more difficult to do in a commercial, so you need to be extremely attentive on the set.

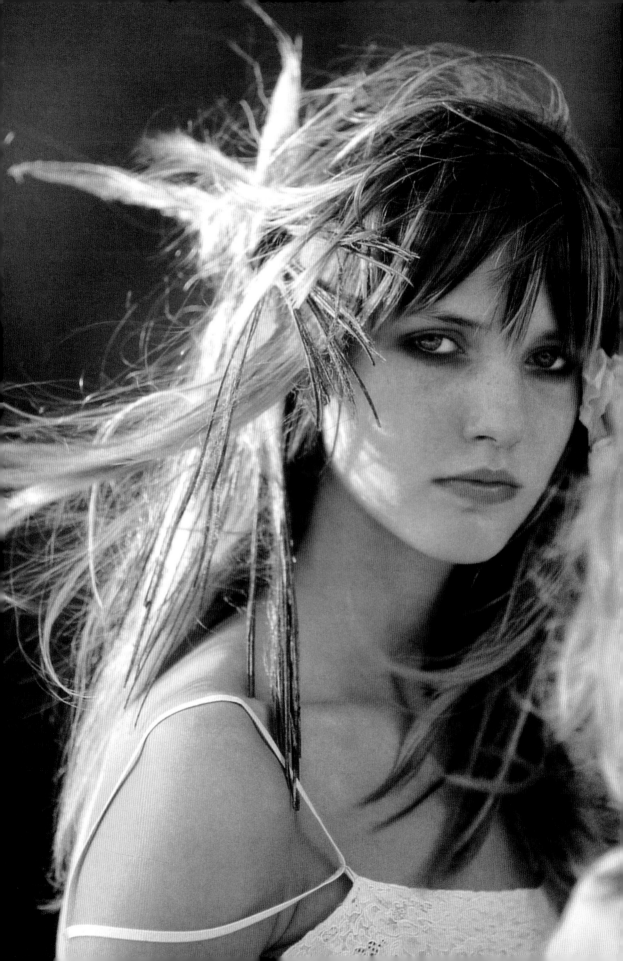

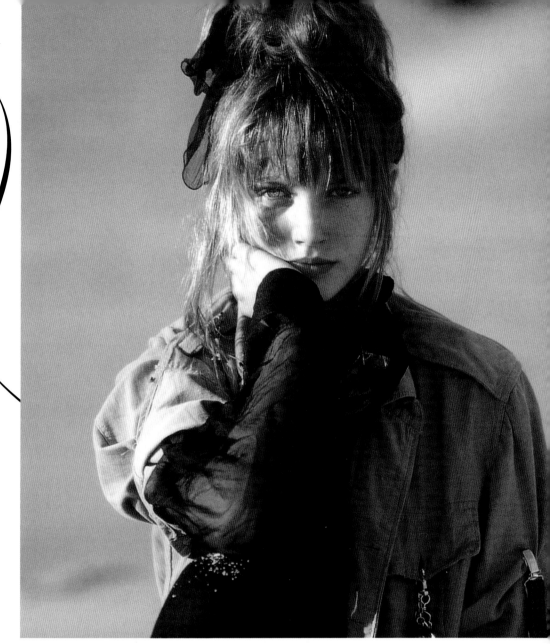

For this fashion shoot, I never did the freestyle makeup the same way twice. *Photos (both pages) by Hans Feurer. Model: Cecilia Chancellor in the Seychelles for French* ELLE. *Stylist: Caroline Baker.*

Both beauty and fashion advertisements (catalogues such as J. Crew and Victoria's Secret) are usually completed over a period of a few days or sometimes a couple of weeks, depending on how many photos are necessary. You usually have several models to make up, and you can usually change the makeup for every new outfit being photographed. Catalogue shoots pay more than magazine editorials but less than television commercials and product ads. Sometimes, catalogue work is less structured than other commercial work, and it can give you more creative freedom, but more often (usually, in fact) it is intense. Lots of different photos must be shot every day. It can be fun, but you can burn out very easily doing too many catalogues. As with any artistic endeavor, you have to be able to bring freshness and creativity to your work to do it well.

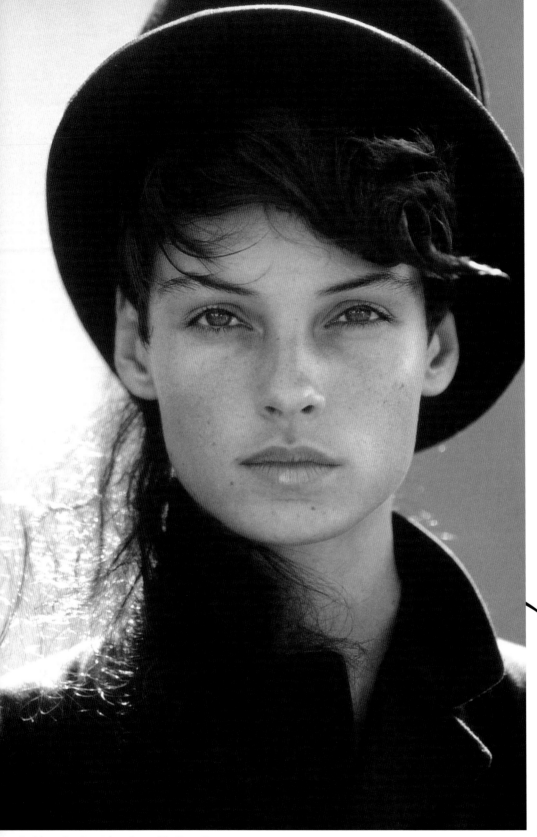

Fashion shoots on location with Hans Feurer. *Photo by Hans Feurer for Italian Vogue, 1986. Model: Famke Janssen.*

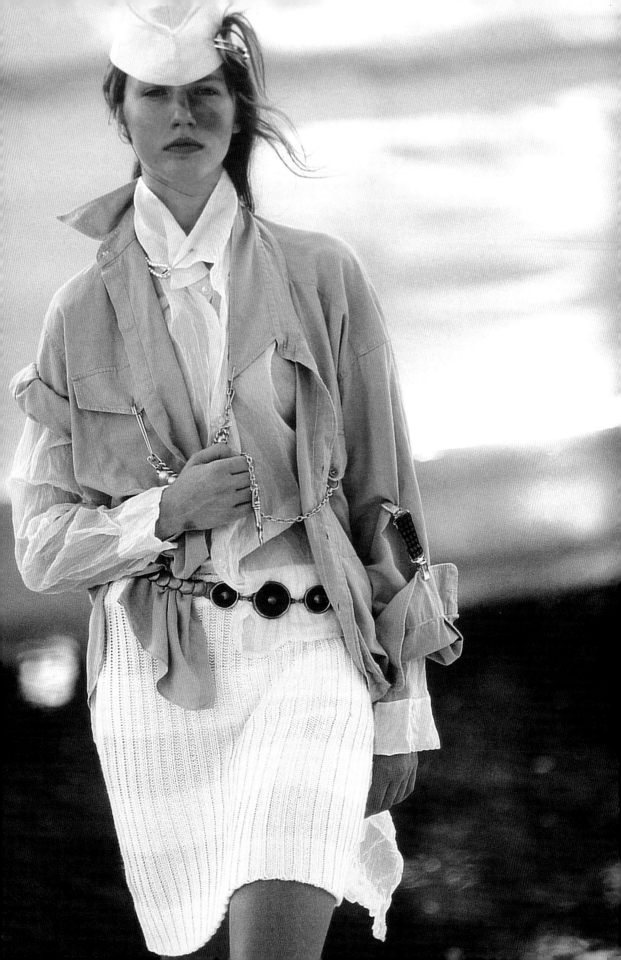

makeup for brides

When you are chosen by the bride to do her makeup, you become part of the most important day of her life. A wedding environment is full of family and loved ones, and you will be chosen to be part of this not only for your makeup talents but also for your contribution to that environment. You must develop the bride's trust from the moment your first contact is initiated. The wedding preparations are stressful, but usually, the time right before the wedding is a wonderful and exciting one. The bride is surrounded by her closest friends and family, all of whom are trying to assist her.

When I first started making up brides other than for a photo shoot, the bride would just book me for the wedding without a trial makeup, and everything would turn out fine. Now it's rare that I do a wedding without first doing a test. However, the test should never be done too prematurely.

Once the bride has decided on both her own and her bridesmaid's dresses for the wedding, as well as her hair color and style, she is then ready to see you. When looking for a word to describe the difference between a bridal makeup and other kinds of makeup a makeup artist may do, I came up with "timeless." Remember, this is a day when the bride wants to look and feel more *beautiful and radiant* than ever before—she will want to look perfect. Every asset she has should be enhanced, even if she just wants her makeup to be "natural" and "clean."

On the day of the test, ask the bride to bring pictures of her dress so you can get a feeling for the type of bride she is going to be. Is it a simple dress? Sophisticated? Romantic? This will help you when making a decision about the style of makeup.

Note for the Bride If you want to use a top-level makeup artist, look in magazines. The agency that the makeup artist works for is usually credited, and you can look up the agency's number, and then call them to try to book the artist. To secure a top artist, you have to be prepared to pay their advertising day-rate and most probably a 50 percent deposit (unless they know you). You should book them six months in advance. Before you get scared off by the potential cost, consider that there are many, many great makeup artists out there who work for considerably less, and there are many ways of working things out within a budget.

Decide how much you have in your budget for a makeup artist and ask around for recommendations. You may find someone who works at your hair salon who is good and whose charge is very reasonable. If you go to a salon instead of having someone come to you to do your makeup, it will be less expensive. You could also book a makeup artist who charges a per-person rate and arrange to have him or her make up a few people so that he or she can earn a reasonable amount.

Discuss money in the very beginning. If you are doing a test, then the price of the test should be discussed, too. The charge for a test is usually about the same as the charge for a makeup lesson (the artist will be spending at least 1 to 2 hours with you). There is usually no fee for a consultation when you meet the artist to look at their portfolio and discuss the makeup, but confirm that there will not be a fee for this when you speak with them or their agent on the phone. Payment is usually made on the day of the wedding, although some artists like to be paid 50 percent in advance.

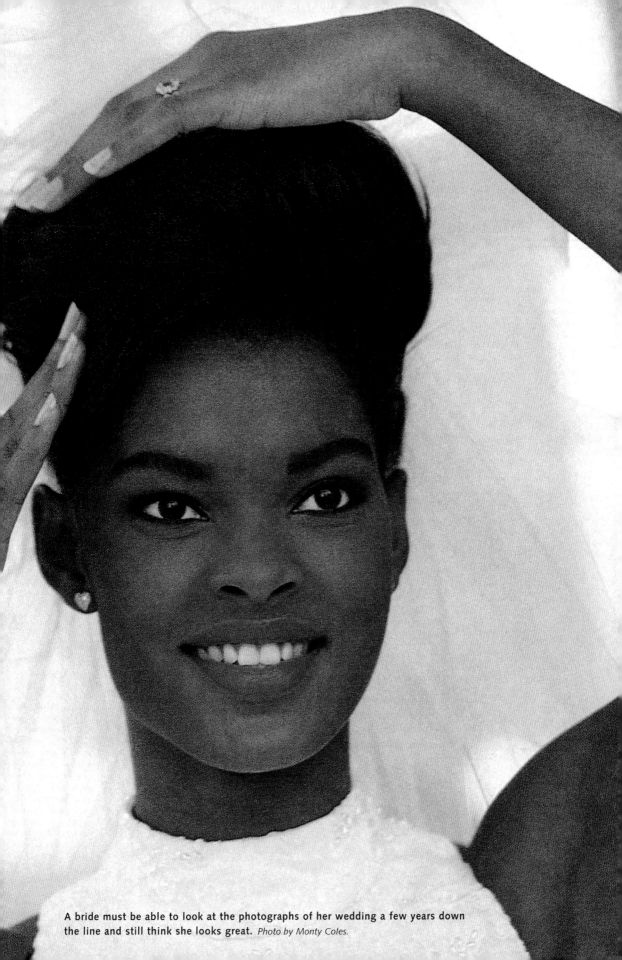

A bride must be able to look at the photographs of her wedding a few years down the line and still think she looks great. *Photo by Monty Coles.*

The time of day at which the wedding is held is also a factor when doing bridal makeup. Evening weddings require a more elegant face, with perhaps a smoky eye makeup, whereas an outdoor, daytime wedding needs a fresher, lighter makeup, especially if wedding photos are going to be taken in the late morning, when the sun is climbing high in the sky. Also, take into account that fact that the bride may not be used to wearing makeup at all, and thus may be overly cautious when you try to experiment on her. You need to work within her comfort level—she will be nervous enough already.

If you've been working doing studio or freelance work, chances are you have a working portfolio. You can show this to the bride in the beginning of the test session or at the consultation. Also, compiling pictures of weddings you've already done is helpful. If you do not have a portfolio, make one with tear sheets that show a variety of looks from different magazines. The client can flip through these pictures and choose a style she likes. Of course, you can elaborate and adapt the looks according to her wishes.

Listen to the bride's likes and dislikes. When looking at the portfolio, make a note of whatever she says she likes, and this will help you get a better understanding of her makeup vocabulary. For instance, I had a client who thought Sophia Loren's makeup was "natural."

When doing a bride's test makeup or consultation, there are a few key issues you need to address with her that could affect the makeup. Is she going on vacation before the wedding or planning on having tanning sessions or using self-tanner? If so you will need to create warmer makeup for her face. Is she having a facial before the ceremony? If so, make sure she doesn't do it the day before the wedding and that she goes to a facialist she has used before to avoid having red, peeling, or irritated skin.

Bridesmaids Some brides also want their bridesmaids' makeup to be applied by a makeup artist.

If you are going to do the bridesmaids' makeup in addition to the bride's, take into account how long it will take.

Knowing where the bridesmaids will be standing during the ceremony in relation to the bride is important. The bride is the queen of the day, and she should receive the most attention. No one else's makeup should compete with hers. If time is limited, have the bridesmaids come wearing their makeup and then adapt it so it looks consistent, appropriate, and so it has a harmonious overall look.

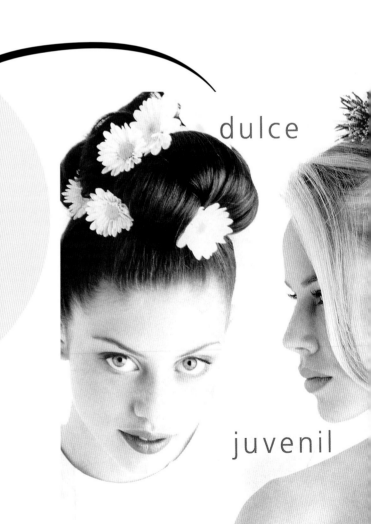

dulce

juvenil

coqueta

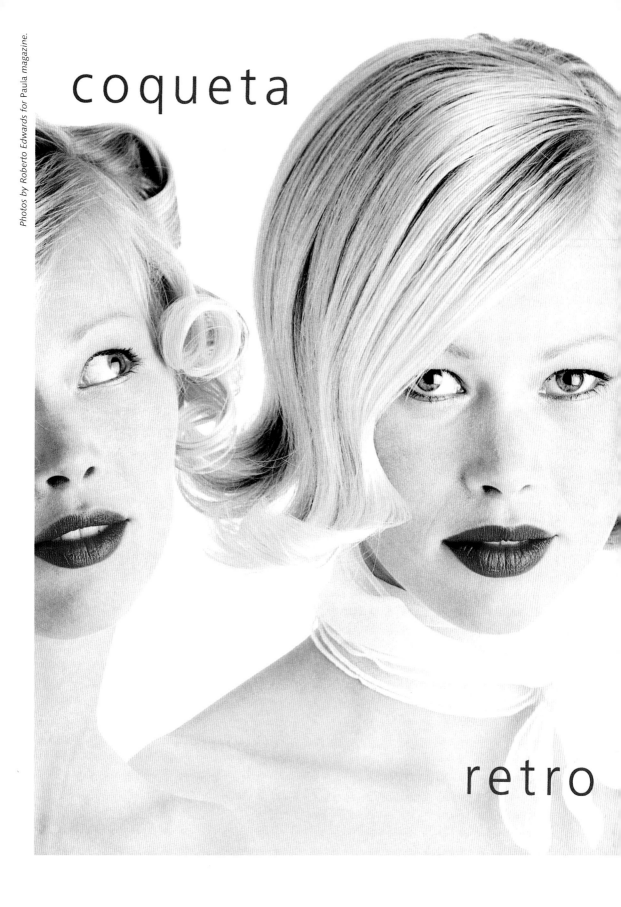

Photos by Roberto Edwards for Paula magazine.

retro

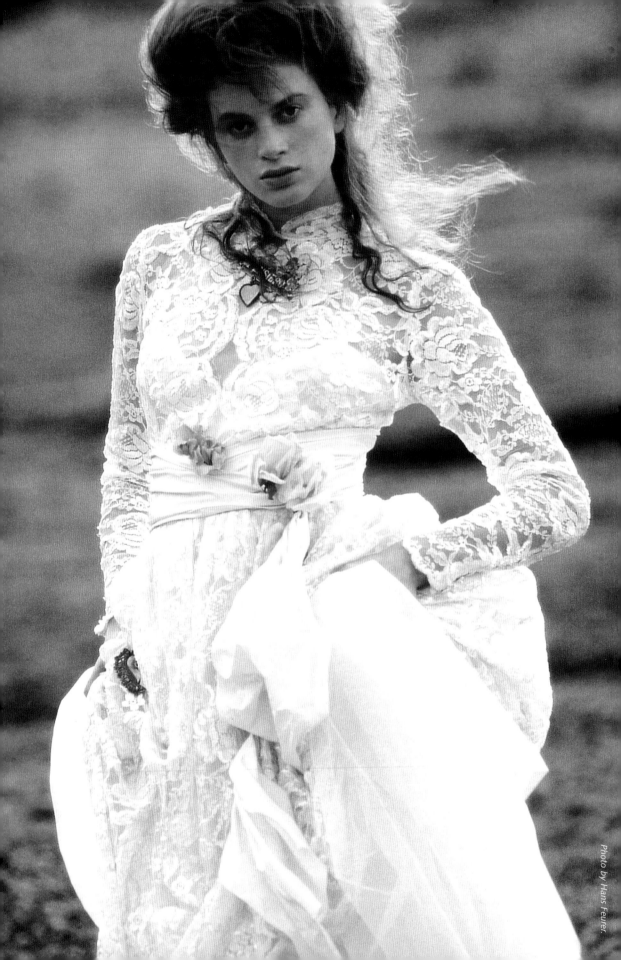

The Wedding Makeup Test

The makeup test is very important. During this time, the bride gets to know you. For the test, the bride should wear something the same color as her wedding dress, or you could drape something around her neck in white or ivory, unless she is planning on wearing a dark color for her wedding.

During the makeup application on the day of the test, don't forget to take notes on what you've done. If you're comfortable with Polaroid cameras, take a picture of the bride. Be aware that Polaroid cameras do not always show true color and texture of makeup.

Try to take the bride a bit further than she would normally go. If she doesn't wear base and has great skin, use just a little concealer. Treat it like a lesson. Start off natural, and strengthen it as you go along. Try a few different lip colors, then try leaving the lips fairly neutral. Change the eyes. If she is going to wear a low-cut dress, then check out her décolletage, neck and shoulders, and back for a difference in the face-to-body color or for any skin imperfections. The face should be only slightly lighter than the body, never darker, which can make it look dull.

Wedding Makeup DON'Ts

- Don't: Line lips too heavily. That can look too harsh. If you insist on lining the lips, soften the edges.

- Don't: Use body makeup over the entire body. Keep it in areas away from the dress, or wipe it down with a tissue once it is applied.

- Don't: Touch the bride's and bridesmaids' dresses while doing the makeup, even if you think your hands are clean.

- Don't: Put too much makeup under the eye.

- Don't: Drink too much champagne.

Wedding Makeup DOs

- Go easy on the foundation, especially on good skin.

- Use touches of "light" for the photos.

- Do a test for the wedding. However, this should never be done too far ahead of time.

- Make sure the bride's face does not look darker than her neck.

- Ask the bride to stop using drying prescription medications such as Retina-A before the wedding.

Fees and Compensation

The time you spend with the bride and at the wedding should be accounted for. You are a professional, and your time is important. The way you charge for wedding makeup is up to you. Some artists charge per person they make up, and some prefer to charge an hourly rate or flat rate.

Understand that it may take you an hour to make up each person, so inform the bride of this. Also, plan to spend much more time on the bride. Plan your day accordingly.

It is good practice for a makeup artist to have set fees for a wedding as they can then be easily recommended to other people. These fees will be affected by many factors. Most important are your notoriety, experience, and the part of the country in which you are situated. In New York or Los Angeles, an artist regularly booked for photo shoots will probably charge the "day rate" that they are paid for an advertising job, which could be in the thousands. The artist knows how important this whole day is to the bride, so he or she should not share it with any other bookings. Depending on how the artist works, he or she may agree to leave immediately upon finishing the makeup, in which case the fee would be less. If a bride hires the artist through an agent, then there will be a 20 percent agency fee added to the total charge. A bride will also be expected to pay for any of the artist's travel expenses and travel time if there is extensive travel involved.

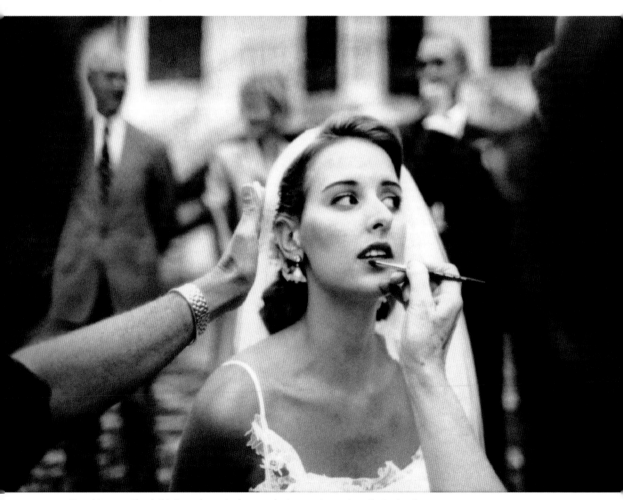

Touching up the bride's makeup before a photo session. *Photo by Frederick Marigoux.*

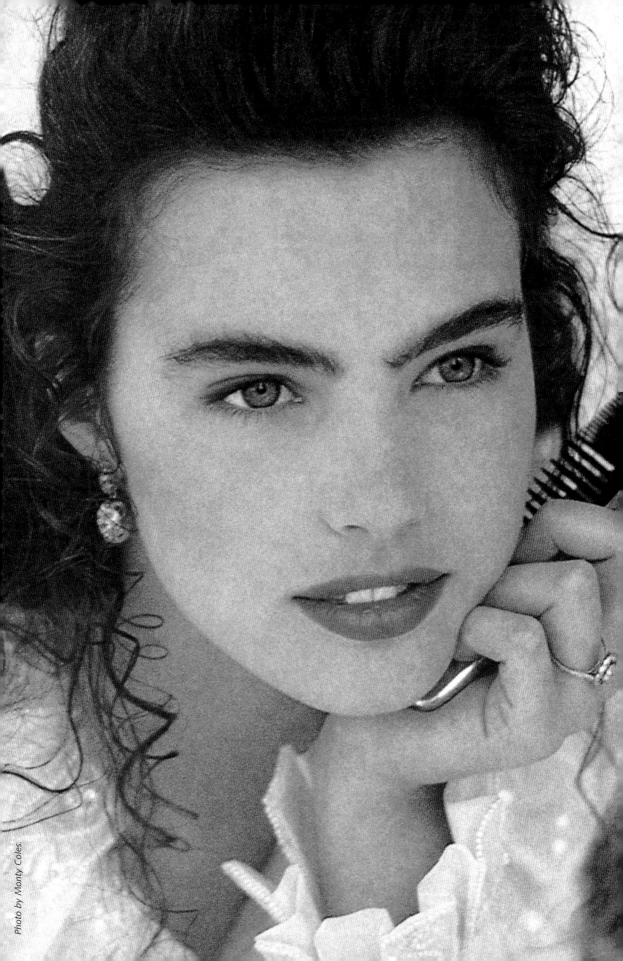

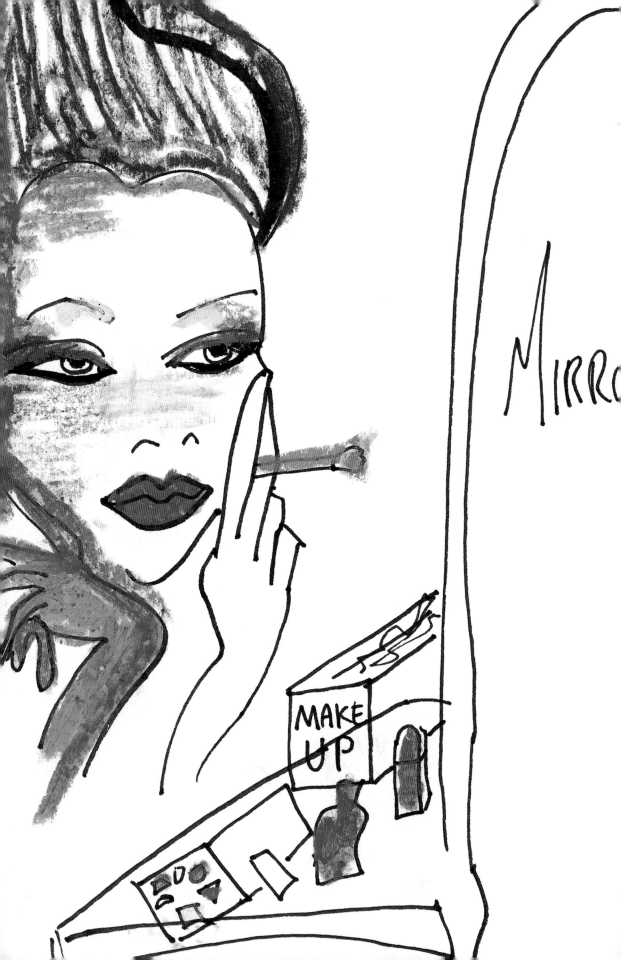

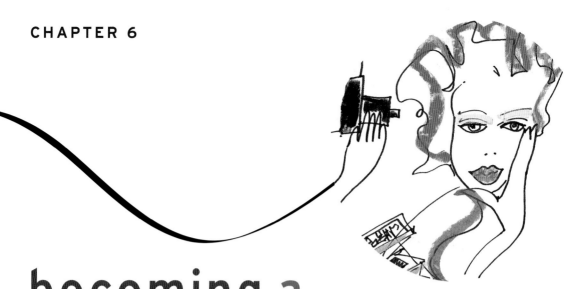

becoming a
makeup artist

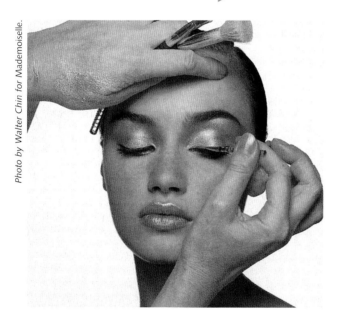

Photo by Walter Chin for Mademoiselle.

I have been asked the question, "How did you begin?" many, many times in my career by aspiring makeup artists. My answer is that I worked at everything I undertook to the best of my ability and made choices in my life guided by intuition and passion rather than caution or a desire for security. That's how I found my path.

Most successful makeup artists have an interesting story about how they got started in the business, and while there is no set formula, many of the stories have common threads that indicate that there may be some qualities essential to becoming a success in the field. If you have a love of people, a passion for doing makeup, a dedication to work, and a strong point of view, you already have a lot in common with many of the big names in the business.

Experiment by trying new makeup styles, colors, and textures on yourself.

getting started

It is extremely important for an aspiring makeup artist to practice doing makeup as much as possible. Practice as much as you can on your friends. Taking makeup classes to learn techniques can give you more knowledge and confidence. It will also give you an edge on your competition if you are planning on assisting or becoming an apprentice with a working makeup artist.

Drawing and painting are also excellent ways to strengthen your sense of color and your technical skill; they help you exercise your hands and develop your taste at the same time. If you can supplement your education with art classes, do so, but if that's not possible, just start sketching and putting your rough ideas on paper. Don't worry too much about what your sketches look like; just keep on trying. Before I started working for Helena Rubinstein's cosmetics company, I could not draw or paint. They asked me to illustrate my makeup ideas on paper. I had been good at geometry in school, so I began creating geometrical faces with a ruler and developed my artistic skills from there.

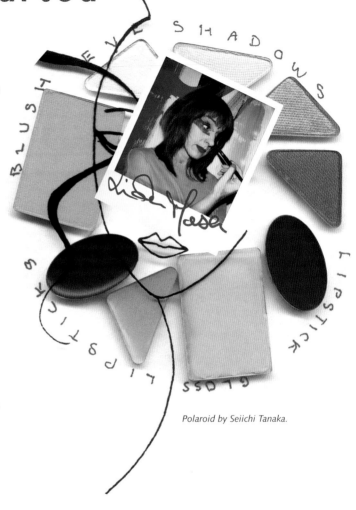

Polaroid by Seiichi Tanaka.

When launching yourself as a freelance makeup artist, maturity is more important than age. One weak link in a team can jeopardize a project and possibly cost a lot of money. Clients and coworkers need to know you can get the job done. They are more apt to trust someone a little older with more experience, but a younger artist with a good attitude and great portfolio can also inspire trust.

I was twenty-eight years old when I began, and being a little older was one of the reasons I felt comfortable with the models; at a younger age, I might have wanted to be in their place being pampered. Twenty-eight was a great age for me to start for other reasons, too. I had pursued other jobs and knew without hesitation that this was my chosen career path. There was nothing I wanted to do more than this, and I had time to free myself from other distractions and devote myself completely to my work.

OPPOSITE PAGE *Contemplation*, Linda Mason, 1999. Acrylic on canvas, 36 x 48 in (91.5 x 122 cm)

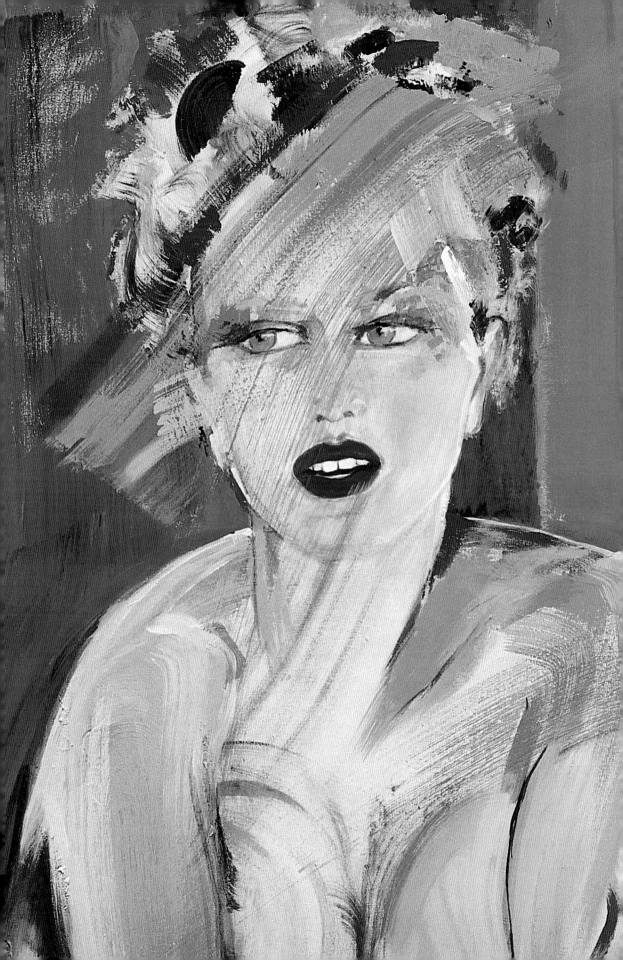

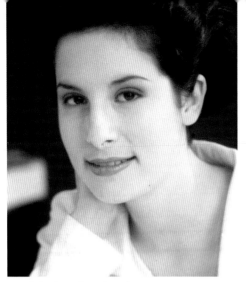

A soft look with nude colors.

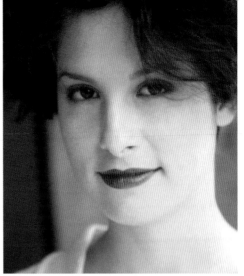

A fun look with earthy colors, brick lip color.

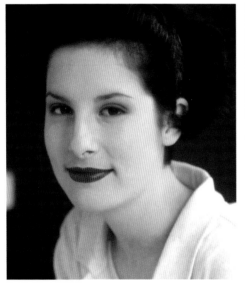

A strong look achieved with deeper brown lips.

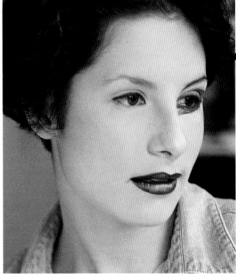

A creative, unconventional look with violet eye and lip color.

Becoming a freelance artist is not the only career path for a makeup artist. Working in the cosmetics department of a retail department store that carries a great variety of cosmetic lines will give any aspiring makeup artist a chance to do what he/she loves, as well as to try out lots of different "goodies" and meet all kinds of people. It could also be the beginning of an important career as a cosmetics company makeup artist, which would be ideal for anyone who needs stability in his/her work. Although working as a freelance makeup artist in fashion and beauty seems very glamorous, it is not for everyone. If the instability of not knowing when and where you will be working next does not appeal to you, then you should consider working for either a department store in the cosmetics department or for a cosmetics company. I trained with and worked for Lancôme for a few years before I became a freelance makeup artist, and doing so was great training.

You can also build up a very good business working in a beauty salon developing makeup not only for special events and proms but also for weddings. You may decide to go into film or television; there are many opportunities in these fields. Be open-minded. You are foremost an artist, and the process of expressing an artistic vision is an adventure!

testing

To get jobs, freelance photographers, models, and makeup artists need a portfolio (their résumé, in effect) that shows examples of their work. The only way to build one when you're starting out is by participating in a "test," a photo shoot based on a makeup, hair, or fashion idea. With luck, the test will result in an interesting photo you can use in your portfolio. You don't have to pay to participate in this type of test because everyone involved is doing so to build his or her portfolio; your makeup, time and talent are what you bring to the table. Testing, most often organized by a photographer, is one of the most exciting opportunities for a makeup artist. It gives you a chance to take all the time you need to experiment with a look and to discover the enjoyment of being part of a team with other people in the industry.

Unconventional, soft and feminine. I strove to retain the beautiful transparency of Suzanna's skin by applying touches of a perfectly matched base only to the imperfections. Mascara and eyeliner can harden the expression, so I used a very delicate, lightly colored eyeshadow and defined the brows lightly with a gold pencil. I defined the natural shape of the lip by applying violet lipstick with a lipbrush, making sure not to go outside the natural lip line.

Actress: Suzanna Midnight. Hair: Cynthia for John Sahag,

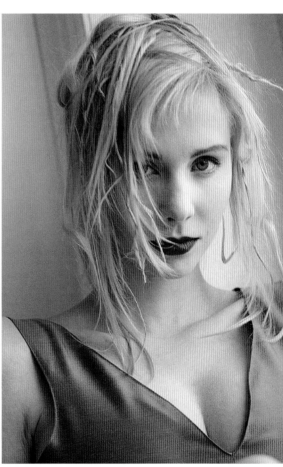

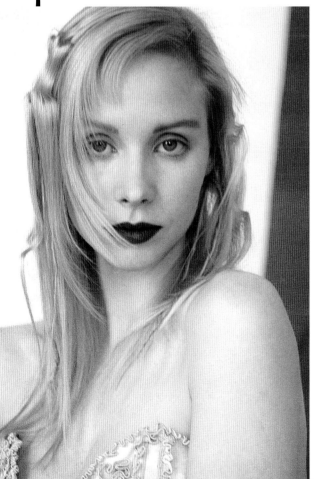

A sultry look with a soft eye and ruby lips. A change in seemingly small things like mascara and the shade of lipstick can make an enormous difference in the atmosphere of the photo.

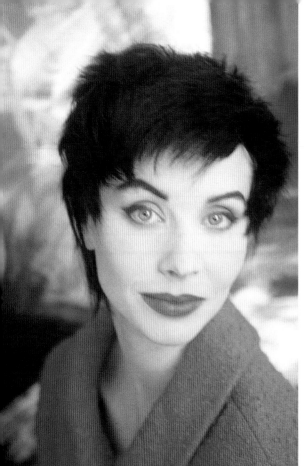

Glamorous, sexy Suzanna in cream base and powder. If the eyes and lips are this intense, it is safer to stay neutral on the cheeks. I used a soft, matte brown shade under the cheekbone. It's useful to practice doing lip shapes with a good red lipstick. I had decided that enlarging the lips would make an enormous difference to Suzanna's face, so before I did her eye makeup, I drew in her lips with a red pencil. After sweeping on gray and brown eyeshadow on the eyelids, I used black eyeliner, mascara, and applied false eyelashes.

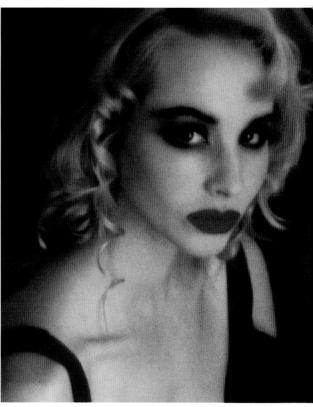

Suzanna again, this time fresh and quirky and wearing a wig. I used a pale base and transparent powder. After applying blue eyeshadow, I lined the eyes with blue cake-liner, which I extended beyond the eye. I then applied lots of black mascara. I defined the brows by strengthening the shape with a brown shade of pencil, then working in a little black to go with the dark hair. Last, I applied a touch of a soft blush and used a soft, natural, berry shade on the lips.

When you do testing work, there are no time constraints or clients to satisfy. You can take as much time as you need to do the makeup. Every time you test, make a point of trying something new so that you can learn through trial and error. In all other respects, treat the test as you would a job. Be professional, always arrive on time, and prepare your makeup and tools as soon as you arrive. Have an idea of what you would like to do, even if you change your mind once you get there. It is good to work with the same model more than once so that you are able to appreciate the different appearances you are able to create on the same face. On my first few tests, I found myself taking at least two to three hours for one "makeup creation"; expect that you'll need to take some time to get it right. Focus on your skills and get the job done to your satisfaction. The most important challenge is to alter the face you are working on without drowning its features; you must also strive to blend the model's look with the theme of the photo shoot.

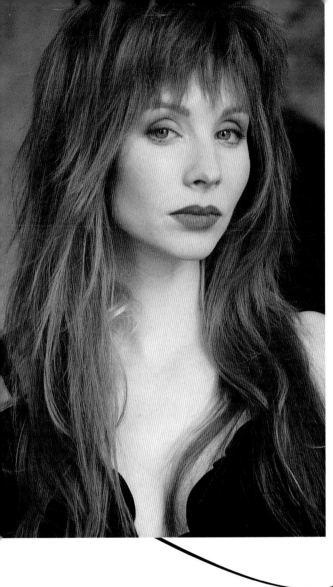

Suzanna as a natural sophisticate. No base. I blended a little brown pencil into the base of the upper lashes, making it stronger in the outer corner of the eye. Then I used an ivory eyeshadow shade over the entire eyelid and a matte, yellow-toned brown sparingly over the pencil in the outer corner of the eye and in the crease. A russet cream-blush was then blended over the apples of the cheeks for freshness. Defining the lips in a warm lip color was the final touch of sophistication.

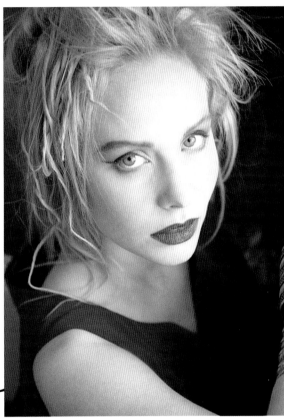

Very light base and lots of powder to pale the skin and make the effect of the colors on the lids stronger. Violet liner over yellow, orange, and violet eye shadows. Deep pink lips.

Start getting your makeup kit together, but don't worry too much about things you don't have. Work with the products you've already got, and to learn to use them effectively. Experiment with the different brushes you have to discover which you prefer and which work better with certain products. Introduce new products and tools to your kit from time to time.

Approach each test with an open mind; put aside all your preconceived ideas about beauty. Somebody seemingly ordinary- or plain-looking could end up making the best photo in your whole portfolio, so treat everyone you make up with that in mind. Ask for the model's input: You can learn from her. However, do not let her *tell* you what to do. Control the situation; this is *your* time to discover your talents. You do not want to do anything out of fear of not being liked or the need to make people happy.

Working with the Photographers

It's often a good idea to meet with the other artists involved in the test beforehand to discuss ideas. The artists pay for their own supplies and materials, and the photographer gives slides or prints of the test to the artists and models involved after reviewing them. Find out whether the photographer is using black-and-white or color film. Colors such as yellow, green, and blue will tend to appear flat in black-and-white film. Using a lighter base and deep shades of red around the eyes will create more depth and contrast in black-and-white film.

It takes more than one testing session to reap benefits, so it is important not to give up on a photographer after one session because you were not satisfied with the initial results. *Building a beneficial working relationship takes time.* Try to make your makeup work better within the context of the photos. Give the photographer feedback, but don't be judgmental. Taste is a difficult thing to assess, but you and the photographer don't have to have the same taste to make the pictures work. You must pin the photographer down a few days after your test to go over the results while everything is fresh in his or her mind, otherwise you will have difficulty. The photographer should give you either slides or prints from your test. You do not need many; just make sure those you get are good shots. A good shot in which it's hard to see the makeup clearly is better than a bad shot in which the makeup looks great.

When I started, I tested with Sammy Georges for a number of months. Then he eventually hired me for all his work, so during my testing period, I slowly moved into the work market. My portfolio grew, and I was able to solicit other photographers to work with me. As his or her career progresses, a makeup artist will gradually fall into a pattern of regular testing with a small group of photographers and thereby build a great portfolio. But this is only possible if one is *always available*, and I don't mean just physically; an artist must always be mentally attentive on the shoot. If one day a photographer decides he wants to test that same night by moonlight in Central Park, you must be available and ready to provide ideas. In the early stages of your career, it's helpful to have a flexible schedule and to have as few other obligations in your life as possible that may interfere with work opportunities that may arise with very little notice.

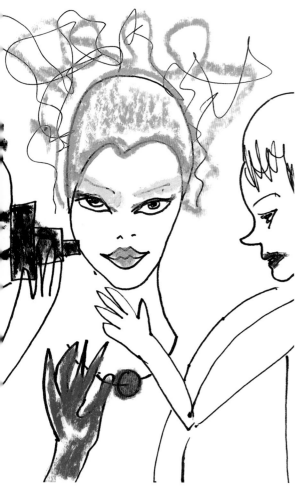

Some photographers don't like you to touch up models' makeup frequently.

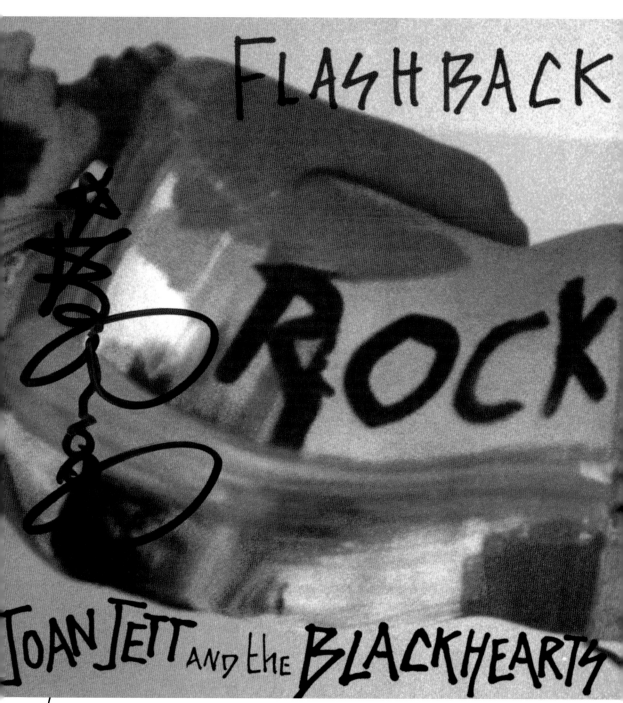

FLASHBACK

ROCK

JOAN JETT AND the BLACKHEARTS

This photo was first used as a makeup test shot that I suggested. Joan Jett ended up using it as the cover for her album *Flashback*.

your portfolio

When you do testing with working photographers, if they see that you are talented, they will gradually gain confidence in you and hire you for paying jobs. Then the clients for whom they are working will probably want to see your portfolio. If the photographers you test with are not in a position to give you paid work, you will still need a portfolio. The more you test, the more confidence you'll gain, and the more antsy you will be to get out there and really do your thing.

A portfolio is basically a collection of photographs and samples of your work that potential clients can review to get an idea of the scope of your talents. You could have only one picture and it might get you work, or you could have twenty-five high-quality pictures, or perhaps just some Polaroids like Kevin Aucoin had in his portfolio when he started. Each person's presentation is different. Don't put a picture you don't like in your portfolio, and don't include a bad photograph because it shows the makeup well. You will be judged on the quality of the photograph more than on the makeup. It's better to have a great picture in your portfolio that doesn't show the makeup (don't go so far as to use a shot that cuts off the model's head) than a bad photo that shows a great face of makeup. Only the client's hairstylist and the makeup artist will dissect the photo and say either "I like the hair" or "I like the makeup"; other people just look and say, "Great photo!" or "Bad photo!" Too many people come to me with a great portfolio jacket with nothing inside it that shows any sense of adventure or style. Don't make the outside of your portfolio distracting. A simple cover is best; focus on the quality of what's inside.

How do you distinguish a good photo from a bad one? Ask for opinions from people whose taste you respect. Don't place too much importance on input from your friends, who may feel compelled to offer support rather than be brutally honest.

The photos in your portfolio are an extension of your style and taste. When I arrived in New York with my portfolio, I was told I would never get work unless I changed it; however, people remembered me because of my portfolio and later offered me creative work. The strength of my portfolio definitely contributed to my success.

One of my
own portfolios.

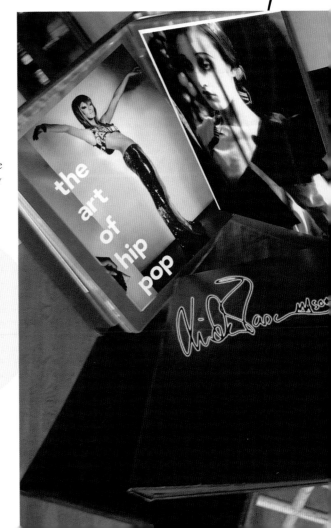

158

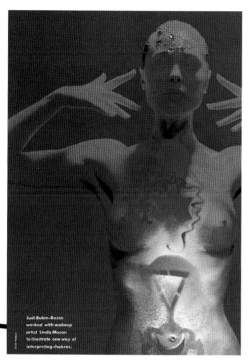

Judi Rubin-Basco worked with makeup artist Linda Mason to illustrate one way of interpreting chakras.

The photographer Jessie Frohman booked me for this magazine article about chakras.
Photo by Jessie Frohman.

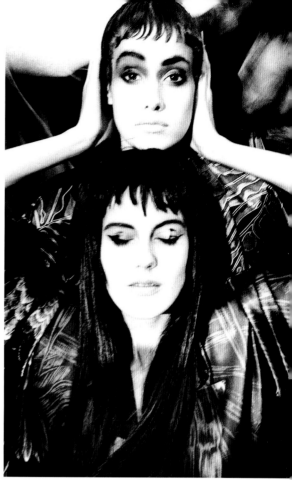

On location in Rome for a Yohji Yamamoto clothing-catalogue shoot. *Photo by Max Vadukul, 1985.*

It's better to have slides from which you can make quality prints when you're ready to show your work. Unless the photographer you're working with is using print film and that's all you can get, don't make prints immediately. Save your slides and review them. Then, when you have tested a little, choose the strongest slides from which you want to make prints. Do laser prints first. Maybe you'll only want laser prints in your portfolio. It is good idea to have both slides and a page of Polaroids in your portfolio as well. Don't include multiple pictures that are almost identical. Learn how to choose the best. If the picture is badly styled or over-accessorized, crop it so that the makeup is what draws the viewer's attention. There are many different kinds of clients, and you can't please them all. In the beginning, I recommend that you have work portraying the kind of makeup you love and enjoy doing the most. If this happens to be a clean, natural look, then make sure the makeup is perfect and you show your versatility through working on a variety of different types of models of all coloring. High-quality prints will best show off this type of work. If you have more creative work, clients will also need to see that you can do clean, fresh makeup. Good laser prints can be a great addition to a portfolio, but a client interested in hiring you will need to see some high-quality prints to be able to see best how clean your work is. You will gradually replace these photos with the ideal: tear sheets and an impressive roster of models and photographers.

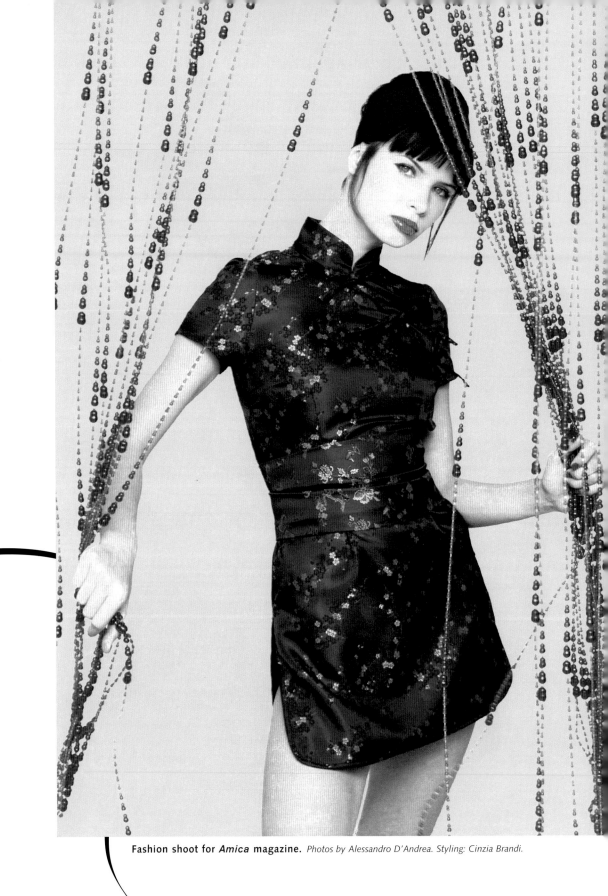

Fashion shoot for *Amica* magazine. *Photos by Alessandro D'Andrea. Styling: Cinzia Brandi.*

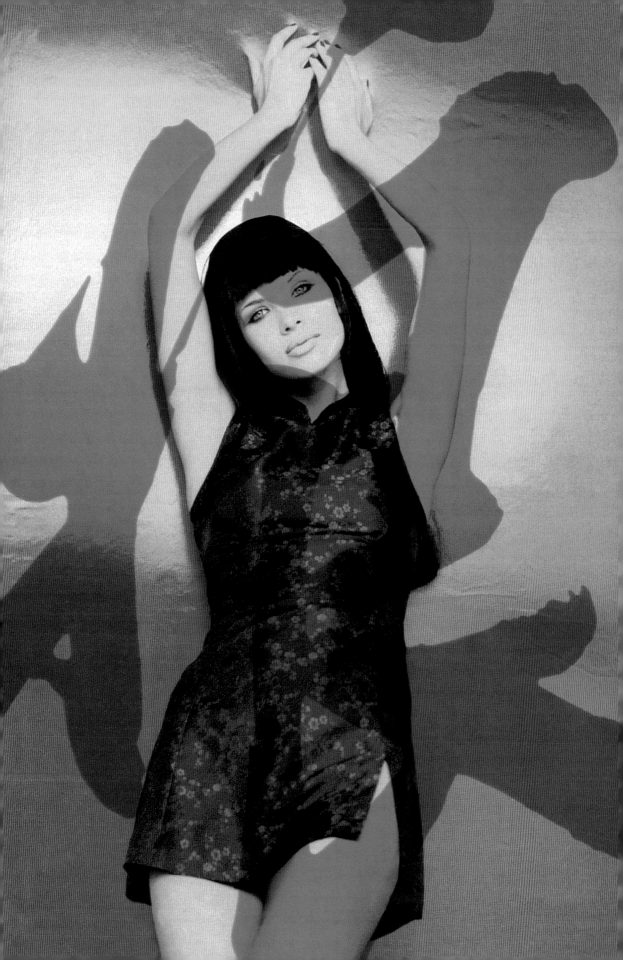

work opportunities

Many makeup artists earn money doing **paid testing** for either model portfolios or composites for actress head shots. Whenever you are asked to do a specific type of makeup for a model or actress portfolio, and the photographer is being paid, you should also receive a fee. You come to an agreement with either the model's agent or the photographer before the testing session about who is to pay you and when. You are often paid by the model at the time of the test. Keep in mind that "paid" testing is a job, and you have to work within certain parameters.

There are some great magazines (such as *Paper*) and Internet sites (such as *ZooZoom.com*) that hire makeup artists for **unpaid editorial work.** They are not able to pay makeup artists and hairstylists, but they will publish your work and allow you to use your full creative ability. Such assignments can be excellent opportunities to experiment and freshen your portfolio with real tear sheets. If you have a makeup idea for a shoot that you would like to see published, you should present it to the editor of such a publication, either in finished form or as a rough idea.

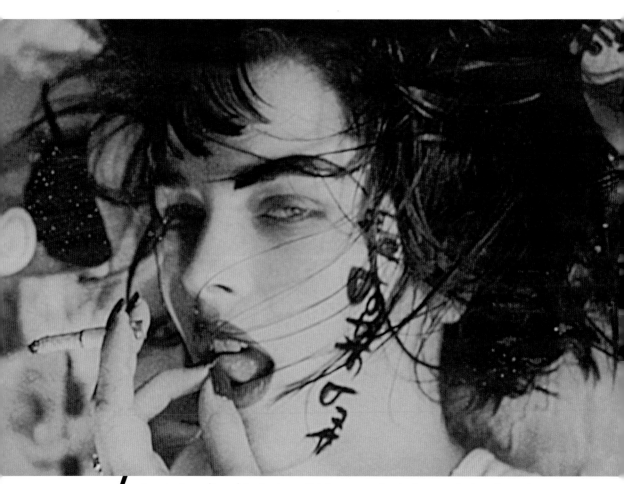

Prosper Assouline of *La Mode en Peinture* magazine in France asked me to work on an idea for them, so I experimented with cinema lighting, food, and terms of endearment written in graffiti on the models' faces and took these photos in 1983.

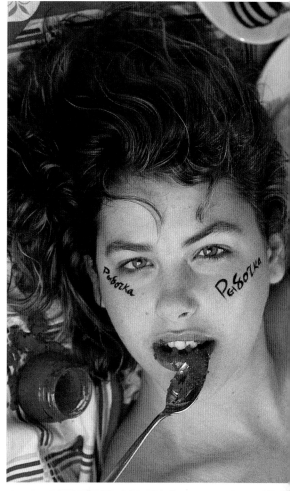
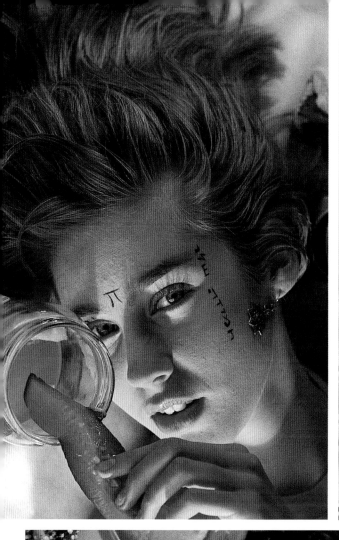
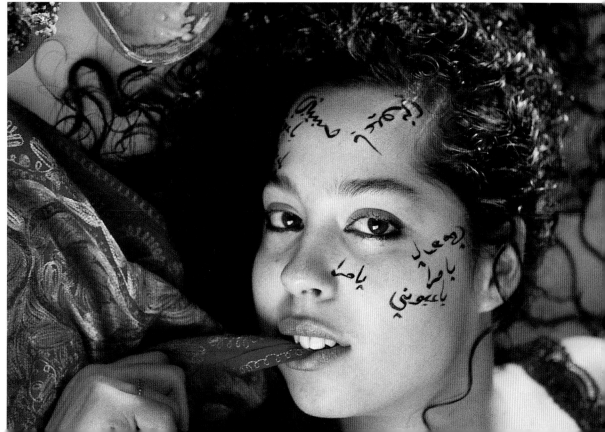

Assisting a Makeup Artist

Assisting an established professional is one of the very best ways to learn the art of makeup. As soon as you have gained that artist's trust, he will start giving you jobs he feels you are capable of doing, which is an excellent way to start working. Makeup artists go through spurts of work, so if you start assisting someone in a slow period, hang in there—you *will* profit from the spurts. When you begin, you won't really be an assistant. You'll be more like an apprentice, and you should not expect to be paid. Assisting is a learning situation, and you must find other ways to be earn money. If the artist for whom you work has a budget for assistants, and you do productive work, then it's possible you will earn something. You may be able to earn just enough money to survive—if you're the kind of person who can live lean with no luxuries. If not, you can find other jobs such as bartending that allow you a flexible schedule so your days are free to assist.

As an assistant, your first duty is to make sure that the makeup artist's kit and tools are clean and organized. Try to remember where things are placed, and if you think of any practical changes you think would be helpful, suggest them first rather than just making them. During the day, ask if anything needs to be washed. Arrange things so that they can be found easily, (for instance, put all the brushes together). Check that pencils are sharpened and burn the points if they need disinfecting. Do not put the material the artist has just used back into the box immediately unless that is where the artist likes to have it while he or she works, but try to make things orderly. Usually artists like to have their tools set out in front of their box. Keep the outsides and tops of bottles clean. Watch what the artist uses so that you know what to take to the set. Always make sure you have tissue and cotton swabs on the set. During the day and at the end of the day, clean the tools and organize the kit. Remember to check the positioning of each article in the kit and how much of each product has been used so you'll know when the artist needs refills.

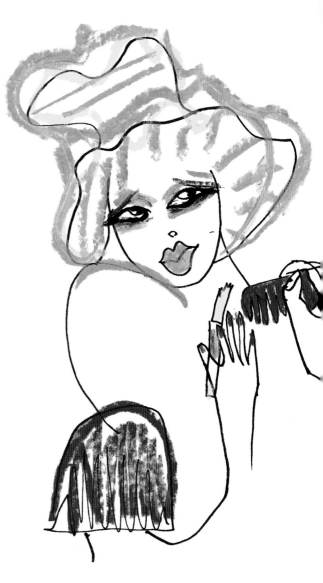

Pay attention and watch discreetly; do not place yourself in too obvious a position. Think about how you would feel first thing in the morning having someone stand staring into your face, doing nothing. Be friendly, but do not talk too much. If the makeup artist and the model are having a conversation, do not interrupt with personal information or draw the conversation to yourself. Keep quiet! Remember, the model must feel special to look special. Do not read magazines, chew gum, or talk on the phone while you are at work. If you're observing or assisting at a photo shoot or a fashion show, do not touch the clothes or try anything on. Be helpful, not only to the artist with whom you are working, but also to the other professionals involved, as long as doing so does not interfere with your principal focus. My first assistant was a textile designer in her twenties, and she did beautiful, stylized drawings. After following me around and learning makeup techniques through observation, she gained quite a few years of experience with detailed artwork, and she quickly made the transition from assistant to makeup artist. Because of the amount of work I was doing and the help I needed for the fashion shows, many of my assistants seemed to make the transition from assistant to makeup artist rather quickly. For their first shows, I just asked them to organize the models, bring them to me to tell them to apply their own base or apply it for them, and to make sure they had the right nail polish on. Thinking back, it was probably about eighteen months before any of my assistants was actually doing full-fledged makeup. I became very irritated with assistants who sat down at shows; I liked them to be *involved* and to look for things to do. If I felt they were good at one thing, I might have them do that one thing over and over on each girl until they had totally perfected whatever it was, such as defining the lips in a certain way. As an assistant, you really have to forget about your ego. Even if you are very good, the makeup artist for whom you are working will still want to put his or her signature on the work. That will means catering your work to express the makeup artist's vision, not your own.

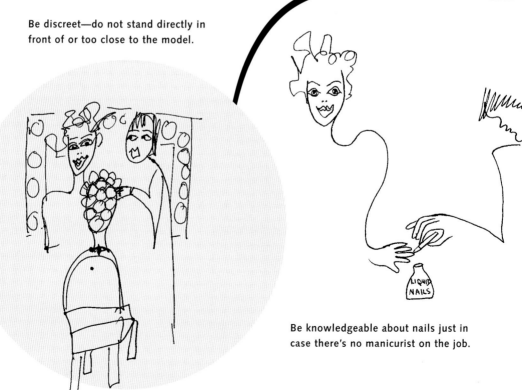

Be discreet—do not stand directly in front of or too close to the model.

Be knowledgeable about nails just in case there's no manicurist on the job.

your makeup kit

Search around for a makeup case. Ask other makeup artists if you can hold their cases to get a feel for their style, size, and organization. Walk with your case. Do you usually run around or take your time getting where you need to go? Do you usually take taxis, a bus, or the subway? Do you have a car? In Paris, I had a very large makeup case, but I had a car and used to drive everywhere or take a taxi. If you are going to be walking a lot with your case, choose one that's portable and suitable for such travel. Cases on wheels are good for taking on buses or the subway, but they aren't suitable for someone like me who often finds herself running to catch trains. I try to find out as much as possible about a job beforehand, and if I need more material than what I normally have in my case, I bring extra bags and boxes and take a taxi to the location. You will probably have quite a few different cases throughout your career.

Make it a habit to:

- Always wash your hands before beginning a makeup and after coughing or sneezing.

- Use spatulas to remove base and other materials from jars.

- Use clean brushes on each model. Have several lip brushes available, or clean the few you have with brush cleaner or 99 percent alcohol.

- Use disposable mascara wands.

- Make sure your sponges, puffs, and so on are immaculately clean.

This Fiberbilt box is, in my opinion, still one of the most practical boxes in existence, but definitely not one of the most glamourous. It is lightweight, strong, incredibly well made, and easy to organize.

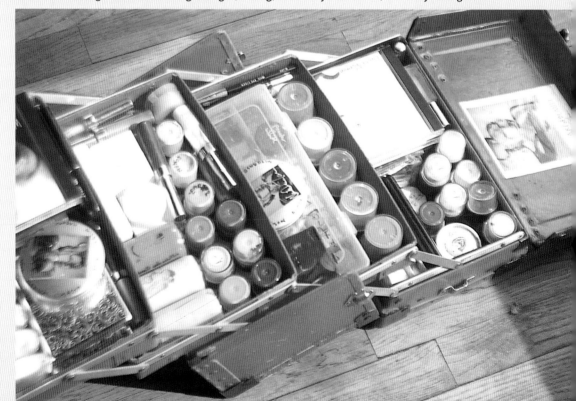

Essentials for Your Makeup Kit

The makeup products and tools in this list are basics for a makeup artist. Color preferences range from artist to artist—after all, part of the enjoyment of being a makeup artist is exploring and using new products. As you go along, you will probably find many products you want to add to your kit. Include water-based, lightweight, liquid foundation in the following ten shades: pale, neutral beige; ivory, medium-light beige; yellow-toned beige; bronze; yellow-toned bronze; brown; white; yellow; very dark brown.

Cream base with heavier coverage (these can be assembled in one compact): three light shades; three dark ones; white; yellow.

Concealer in cream consistency (also good to have these in compact form): light; medium; dark. You can mix the white and yellow cream bases with these if you need to make adjustments.

Loose powder white; yellow tone; brown.

Pressed powder translucent; medium; olive. You can mix both the loose and pressed powder. If in doubt, powder first with the translucent, then powder sparingly with the colored powders. If you are dealing with very pale skin, powder first with white then translucent.

Powder blush soft pink; coral; red; muted pink; brown.

Cream blush pearl; bronze; pink; red; russet.

Eyeliner pencils black; brown; light brown; gray. They should be soft in texture.

Brows pencils blonde; brown; gray; black. These should be hard in texture.

Liquid or cake liner black; brown.

Eye shadows Matte: white; ivory; gray; brown; black; peach; blue; green; yellow; violet. **Pearl:** white; beige; pink; lilac. **Cream:** yellow; blue; red.

Mascara brown; black.

Lip pencils brown; nude; soft, muted pink; soft cherry red.

Lipsticks It is good to have a palette with choices for mixing colors. Make a pale beige by mixing nude and brown. White pearl mixed in with any color will make it pearlized. Pure, bright hues such as pink, orange, violet, and red can be used pure and bright as stains, or added to nude or brown to make muted lip shades.

Lip gloss

False eyelashes black and brown individual clusters in long, medium, and short; four pairs of eyelashes in strips (two black pairs and two brown pairs); lightweight and heavy.

Cleanser, toner, and **moisturizer** for sensitive skin with no perfumes added.

Almond oil for facial massage and care.

Eye makeup remover non-oily.

Tools, brushes, and **sponges** A collection of the tools and brushes shown throughout the book will be ample for you to begin with. You will, however, need more sponges, powder puffs, disposable mascara wands, and some disposable lip brushes.

Miscellaneous Cotton swabs, tissues, pencil sharpener, small scissors, eyelash curler, eye drops, glycerin, eyelash glue, 99% alcohol, hand sanitizer.

Always strive to keep your makeup kit as immaculate and organized as possible. Arrive on the job with the kit clean and in order, otherwise you will create a bad impression when you open it. Always observe the following general rules for keeping your equipment sanitary.

- Wash your brushes with hot water and soap *after every session* by rubbing them on a bar of soap, then rubbing the hairs together between your fingertips. Rinse thoroughly. They should be squeaky clean; disinfect them by immersing them in alcohol. Do not rub them dry on a towel because this will spread the hairs. Squeeze them gently with a paper towel, let them finish drying naturally.

- Keep your kit organized, and set out what you think you'll need in an orderly fashion when you arrive at your destination. Try as best you can to organize it again and clean everything before you close your kit at the end of your session. Your makeup box is a reflection of who you are and the respect you have for the person on whom you are work. You never want to appear haphazard or sloppy.

- Disinfect tweezers with alcohol.

- Burn and sharpen the points of your pencils between use on each model.

- To avoid irritating skin or provoking allergies, use non-oily eye makeup remover and non-perfumed natural cleansers and moisturizers.

This Leichner box I bought in Paris and spray-painted myself was my favorite box of all time. It was narrow and therefore comfortable for carrying by my side. It held a lot and was also elegant.

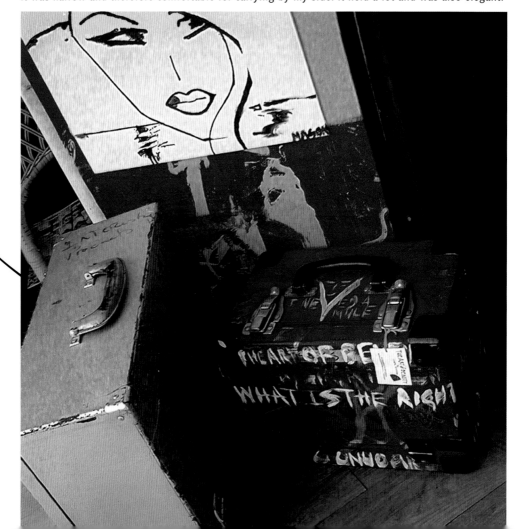

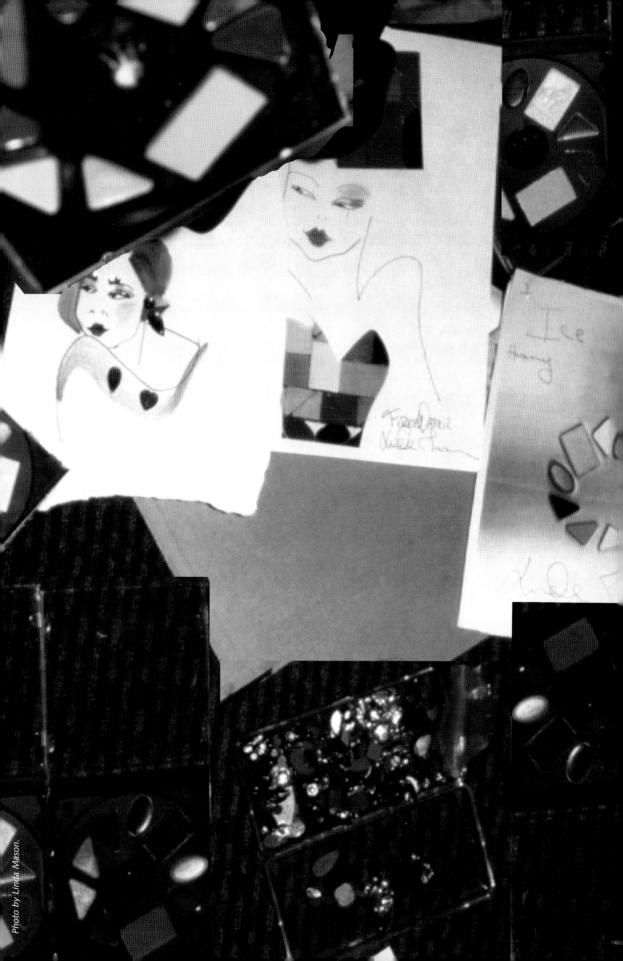

resources

Courses/Schools

EAST COAST

New York

IL MAKIAGE   107 East 60th St., NY, NY, 10022

Phone: 212-371-3992

www.il-makiage.com

Offers a wide range of courses in the study of makeup. The courses are taught like a science course, with detailed charts, slides, and lectures by makeup professors. Tools and products are provided for each student in every session, including a set of professional brushes and a 25 percent product discount, and inclusion in the Il Makiage global referral database.

LIA SCHORR INSTITUTE   686 Lexington Ave., NY, NY, 10022

Phone: 212-486-9541

www.liaschorrinstitute.com

This skin-care training institute offers students the opportunity to train with Lia Schorr, a top skin-care practitioner. Students will learn how to use state-of-the-art equipment and earn the hours they need to get their state aesthetician's license. There are seven major classes, ranging from aesthetiques, advanced aesthetiques, advanced waxing, electrolysis, basic makeup, bridal makeup, theatrical makeup, and a preparatory course for the aestheticians examination. The complete aesthetiques course requires 600 hours of class training.

THE ART OF BEAUTY BY LINDA MASON   26 Grand St., NY, NY, 10013

Phone: 212-625-0490; Fax: 212-716-1114

www.lindamason.com

Linda Mason offers an intensive seven-course certificate program for any level artist on makeup application for runway, fashion, beauty, and brides. An industry veteran, Linda bombards you with knowledge, then throws you in at the deep end to exercise your talents. A live photo-shoot is conducted to provide hands-on experience and to give each student a professional photo for his or her portfolio. Classes are held in Linda Mason's studio and taught by Mason herself, a world-renowned celebrity makeup artist.

DEBRA MACKI COSMETICS

Phone: 800-463-3272

www.debramacki.com

Boston-based makeup artist Debra Macki is the official makeup czar of New England. With her own line of cosmetics and staff of studio makeup artists, she established her company to reflect her easygoing personality. Macki prefers to keep her classes fun. They are taught by one of the studio makeup artists and are given in Atlanta, Georgia; Boston, Massachusetts; Chicago, Illinois; San Diego, California; San Francisco, California; and Miami, Florida. Visit the company web site for locations and schedules.

North Carolina

LEON'S BEAUTY SCHOOL

www.leonsstylesalons.com/school/

Leon's Beauty School has been training students in the southeast for over 30 years. The school is licensed by the North Carolina State Board of Cosmetology Art Examiners and is fully accredited by the National Accrediting Commision of Cosmetology Arts and Sciences. They offer courses in both cosmetology and esthetiques. Their goal is to "educate [their] students in marketable cosmetology skills which enable graduates to find profitable employment."

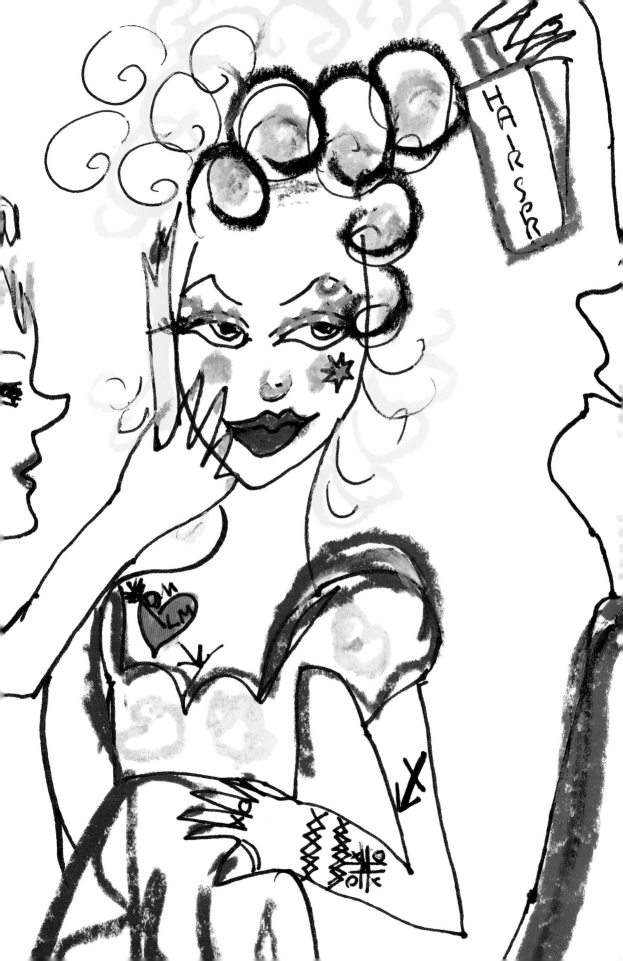

California

CINEMA MAKEUP SCHOOL 3770 Wilshire Boulevard, Los Angeles, CA, 90010

Phone: 213-368-1234

www.cinemamakeup.com

MUD 129 South San Fernando Boulevard, Burbank, CA 91502   375 West Broadway, #202, New York, NY 100012

Phone: 818-729-9420 or 212-925-9250

www.mud.com

Make-up Designory is a private postsecondary institution that provides training every year to hundreds of students from around the world to work in fashion, film, and television. Specialties include beauty makeup artistry, hairstyling, wardrobe, character makeup, and special makeup effects. The school has two locations, one in Los Angeles (founded in 1997) and one in New York (MUD's second facility in the United States).

WESTMORE ACADEMY OF COSMETIC ARTS 916 W. Burbank Blvd., Suite R, Burbank, CA, 91506

Phone: 818-562-6808 or 877-978-6673

www.westmoreacademy.com

The Westmore Academy, founded in 1981 by Marvin Westmore, is a family-owned operation and is part of a Hollywood dynasty that has lasted more than eighty years. The first film studio makeup department was actually created in 1917 by George Westmore. The Westmore Academy offers courses in every aspect of the makeup artistry field: motion picture, photography and fashion, spa salon, and medical. There is a master course for beauty, character, historical, and makeup effects for motion pictures and television. There are master courses for portraiture, fashion, glamour and commercial photography, and a beauty and fashion makeup for spas and salons course. In addition to an in-depth study in art principles, intensive color training, and the psychology of color, included in the 12-week course are sketching, drawing, and sculpting. Students are required to purchase the Westmore Academy makeup kit for their particular course at an additional fee (this ensures that each student has the proper tools).

Texas

ELAN MAKE-UP STUDIO 1921 1/2 Greenville Avenue, Studio B, Dallas, TX 75206

Phone: 214-370-3333

www.elanmakeup.com

Elan Make-up Studio is an educational training center which enhances student's knowledge and skills in all aspects of makeup artistry. We strive to bring out our student's natural talent and desire through our extensive training of makeup techniques and products. the program combines theory, demonstrations, and slides. It is designed to make the student proficient in beauty and corrective techniques in order to further their careers.

Canada

MASTER MIND MAKE-UP ACADEMY 206-2nd Ave North Saskatoon, Saskatchewan S72B5, Canada

Phone: 306-652-2002; Fax 306-652-4351

The primary goal at Master Mind Academy is to provide students with the highest quality education possible and prepare them for employment as makeup artists. The school offer two levels of courses. Level I is for beginners; it allows students to pick up the fundamentals of different applications, color theory, lighting face shapes, tools, supply knowledge, and skin care. Level II is for advanced students who have had at least 36 hours of training in makeup artistry. This class is more in depth, and students learn the art of cosmetics for theater, including special effects such as burns, bruising, old age, latex, scars, etc. There are day and evening classes to choose from. Included in the tuition are books, and a photo shoot (the student must supply the model).

BLANCHE MACDONALD CENTRE 100-555 West 12th Avenue, Vancouver, B.C. Canada V5Z 3X7

Phone: 604-685-0947

www.blanchemacdonald.com

The Blanche Macdonald Centre for Applied Design has been established since 1960. Given that the Makeup program is continously updated and upgraded, the college is adamant about ensuring that their training remains progressive and industry responsive. Spanning ten comprehensive training levels from fundamentals to special makeup effects, the program goes beyond the basic tools and techniques required when working in this dynamic medium. Their interactive classroom experience and educational approach have a reality-based context prepare their students for a prosperous career.

London

DELAMAR ACADEMY OF MAKE-UP Ealing Studios, Building D, Second Floor, Ealing Green, London W5 5EP

Phone: (0) 20.8579.9511

www.TheMake-UpCentre.co.uk

Delmar Academy is for those who are serious about going into film or fashion makeup. Every genre is covered with the same intensity. The period wig class is just as thorough as the facial anatomy class. The teachers are experts in their fields and many are film and fashion veterans. Many graduates have gone on to do notable things in the industry: Graduate Christine Bludell is an Oscar winner (for the makeup in Mike Leigh's film *Topsy-Turvy*). Makeup artistry courses offered cover all areas of the art, from fashion and beauty to prosthetic makeup. Length of full-time courses ranges from 3 months up to the one-year certificate course. All materials and makeup kits are given to 3 month and one-year students. Delamar Academy also offers numerous specialized workshops.

JEMMA KIDD MAKE-UP SCHOOL Garden Studios, 11-15 Betterton Street, London WC2H

Phone: (0) 20.8509.3291

www.jemmakidd.com

The School was set up in 2003 to train professional makeup artists to the highest standard and launch their careers in the industry. The school offers a range of workshops, masterclasses, and one-to-ones. There are only a maximum of fourteen students per group course, so that they can give each student the most hands-on teaching experience.

Paris

JEAN-PIERRE FLEURIMON MAKEUP SCHOOL 274 Rue Saint Honore, 75001, Paris

Phone: 01.42.61.29.15; Fax: 01.42.61.29.75

THE JEAN PIERRE FLEURIMON TRAINING CENTER AND MAKEUP SCHOOL 39 Rue Galilée, 75116, Paris

www.fleurimon.com

The Training Center offers traditional professional courses. The Jean-Pierre Fleurimon Makeup School offers a three-, six-, or nine-month certificate course covering makeup for photography, television, cinema, special effects, theater, and body painting. The courses take place daily, in the mornings and afternoons (you gain double the hours if you compare the program to those of schools that give a choice between either morning or afternoon classes). The fee includes makeup products, including those for special effects and latex masks (these are not always mentioned in the information you receive from the school). A book is given free of charge to students who follow the three-, six- or nine-month courses. The book contains the best photos of students' hands-on makeup applications and serves as a professional reference for each student to use when seeking a job.

Books

Even though you may only wish to do fashion and beauty makeup, it is useful to know about other aspects of the industry and to have a basic knowledge of theatrical and movie makeup. If you do not wish to take classes on those subjects, there are some great books out there that will give you this knowledge. I encourage you to purchase "art" books that inspire you, such as books on artists like Picasso and Van Dongen, or tabletop photography books on fashion or an era like the '50s or '60s.

STAGE MAKEUP by Richard Corson and James Glavan, 9th edition (Allyn & Bacon)

Corson and Glavan's book is one of the more thorough of this genre and is written with the precision of a medical journal. Corson explains his points with drawings, photographs, and several cartoons. There are charts about everything you could think of, from "twentieth-century hair-do's" to "creating a likeness of Woodrow Wilson." This is a practical and comprehensive book that guides you through preparation and basic techniques. Explains how to use shading and highlighting to broaden or thin a face, distort a nose, or hide scars and blemishes. Explains how to plan and execute your makeup for effective characterization. Includes sections on stylized fantasy work, period makeup, and special effects, including extremely lifelike cuts, stitches, black eyes, and bruising.

MAKEUP YOUR MIND by François Nars (Powerhouse Books)

Makeup Your Mind combines cosmetics designer François Nars' two remarkable talents–makeup and photography, both of which he uses to show women how to enhance their natural beauty. It is a comprehensive compilation of before-and-after photographs, with precise instructional guides on clear plastic overlays indicating exactly what goes where, allowing you to see the finished effect for perfect results.

MAKEUP MAKEOVERS: EXPERT SECRETS FOR STUNNING TRANSFORMATIONS

by Robert Jones (Fair Winds Press)

Robert Jones, makeup artist, shows women how to transform themselves by enhancing their natural beauty. No matter what your age, skin tone, or profile, Robert will show you simple techniques that camouflage flaws and highlight each woman's unique beauty.

CREATE YOUR OWN STAGE MAKEUP by Gill Davies (Watson-Guptill Publications)

Create Your own Stage Makeup helps makeup artists create faces for different kinds of roles or performances. The book explains materials, preparation, and application with color illustrations and step-by-step instructions. Covers stage makeup for musicals and ballets, fantasy and animal roles, youth and age, false noses, wounds, beards, and other special effects, and more.

MAKING FACES by Kevin Aucoin (Little Brown & Co.)

Along with Kevin Aucoin's other books *The Art of Makeup* and *Face Forward,* this book is beautiful to have and beautiful to behold. Techniques are lavishly illustrated. This book is excellent for would-be makeup artists or anyone who wants to learn how use makeup well.

Noteworthy

AIR CRAFT COSMETICS

Phone: 323-876-8488

www.aircraftcosmetics.com

Many makeup artists, especially for film, are now using an airbrushing technique. Special foundations have been formulated specifically for this purpose. Air Craft Cosmetics, founded by makeup artists Kris Evans and Emmy award-winning Darla Albright, specializes in this water-based airbrushing base product that has no plasticizers or alcohol. Unlike other airbrush cosmetics, this product allows you to touch it up with a sponge or brush.

THE HOUSE OF PORTFOLIOS CO. INC

52 West 21st Street, New York, NY 10010

Phone: 212-206-7323

www.houseofportfolios.com

Manufacturer and sellers of fine hand-made portfolios. They have been master craftsmen in the custom portfolio industry for over thirty years.

LE BOOK

www.lebook.com

Le Book is the world's first and only trade publication for the fashion, beauty, design, entertainment, publishing, and advertising industries. A great place to find out who represents makeup artists, hairstylists, and photographers.

Le Book London
8-10 Dryden Street, 4th floor
London, WC2E 9NA
Phone: (0) 20.7836.98.88

Le Book New York
552 Broadway, 6th Floor
New York, NY 10012 USA
Phone: 212-334-5252

Le Book Paris
4, Rue D'Enghein
75010 Paris
Phone: 01.47.70.03.30

INDEX